Do You Know Lisa?

Collection of Primary Health Care Articles. Volume 4

Dr. Lisa Goins PhD, APRN, FNP-BC, RMT

Welcome to Volume 4 of *Do You Know Lisa?*

Wow! This is the Volume 4! If you have missed Volumes 1, 2, and 3, the books are located on Amazon.com.

Do you know Lisa? She is your Nurse Practitioner who can answer your questions or find out those answers for you. This book is a collection of articles published on social media sites for the year of 2017, located in print for easy reading, collecting, and resource material. Individuals can follow or submit question to Dr. Lisa via the internet at www.couturehealthcare.org.

Who is this Lisa you speak about?

Dr. Lisa Goins PhD, APRN, FNP-BC, RMT is the CEO and Founder of Couture Health Care, an IRS and US Postal Service recognized 501c3 nonprofit corporation established in 2013. Mission Statement: *"Couturing individual patient's / client's spiritual and health care needs for best outcomes"*

Dr. Goins has worked in the health field since 1989. She has worked as a resident care tech, LPN, RN, RN-ASN, RN-BSN, RN-MSN, and RN-DNPc. Dr. Goins is a Board Certified Family Nurse Practitioner in the State of Ohio, USA since 2012. Dr. Goins holds non-secular Bachelors, Masters, and PhD. Dr. Goins is licensed as Clergy in the State of Ohio and is a Reiki/Master/Teacher.

Dr. Goins' articles may be found on:

www.couturehealthcare.org

Google+, Twitter, LinkedIn, Facebook, and videos on YouTube.

Couture Health Care's office is located on 201 North Brookwood Ave., Hamilton, OH 45013, Telephone 513-857-5679.

In addition to working with Couture Health Care, Dr. Goins works with Dwarven Tavern and Foundation for Spiritual Research.

Dedication:

Thank you to all the patients of Couture Health Care. We hope to see you for another 20 years!

Special thanks to Couture Health Care's staff for doing the impossible with nothing and making the possible every day for our patients.

Ultimate thanks to Couture Health Care's Board Members in believing in a dream and making it a reality.

Disclaimer:

This is the forth volume of health care articles in the collection of *Do You Know Lisa*. The content is designed for education of the public and is generalized. As awesome as the content of this book is, it is not a replacement visit for seeing your Nurse Practitioner.

Information:

Should the material in this book OFFEND thee, then put the book down or give it to someone else.

Editing:

Typos and errors do happen. My apologies in advance. Dr. Lisa views typos and errors as copy rights. Winning!

Thank You:

Thank you for purchasing, downloading, and reading this book. I appreciate your support and may you find the content useful in your daily life. Please follow up and leave a review online. Do share the book with friends and family. Blessings! May your health be excellent, if not, give me or your local Nurse Practitioner a call to schedule a visit.

Why Do I Have to Come Back for a Medication Check?

The provider will see a patient for a visit and may want to try a new medication or increase/decrease a dose. Certain medications need to be monitored so they do not cause the wrong reaction.

Medications of concern are mental health and heart medications that will take some time to take effectiveness before desired effect. This will mean that the patient may need to return sooner than for refills to be evaluated.

At the medication check appointment, the vital signs will be done and blood work or other testing may be done to determine if the medication is agreeing with the patient for the correct results.

Patients that miss these appointments may hinder their health care outcomes and may have important health problems missed until their next appointment. Patients need to return to the appointments regardless of how they feel to be evaluated.

If they feel good the goals may being met and need to be documented. If they feel bad, then there may be changes and documented.

Medication visits are focused visits unlike first visits or refill visits. This visit is all about the medication but other problems may or not be discussed depending on time set aside for the patient. Additional education, reading or review materials may be give, and a referral for a specialist may be discussed.
It is always good to follow up with a medication check when scheduled.

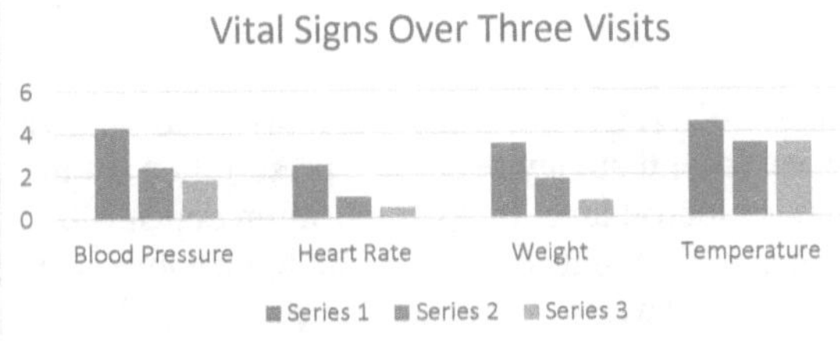

Why Can't I Eat Before Blood Testing?

This visit the patient shows up and the provider wants to get blood work done. What does this mean to the patient? The provider requesting the blood testing will want to get an evaluation of body fluids to discern, if there should be any medication or any changes in medication.

The provider will order blood testing. This means that the provider will check of a list of various blood tests that they want done for the patient. Many times, blood tests may include regular testing such as complete blood count that can tell the provider if there is anything wrong with the cells or a patient is anemic.

Male testing may include a prostate blood test to get a number. This number will tell the provider if the prostate is healthy or a referral to an urologist may be needed. Female hormone testing may allow a patient to confirm they are pregnant or pre-menopause. Additional testing may confirm thyroid, liver, and kidney functions. Specific tests can tell a provider if the patient is having a heart attack or they may have testing criteria results for Lyme's disease.

The provider may then review the results with the patient and confirm any problems or verify health of systems. Lab work may be done on site during a visit or at a location nearby that offers the provider access to expensive machines that would not be financially feasible onsite or specialized testing.

But why can I not eat? Some testing results can change on the day that a patient eats. This can cause skewed results that may result in the patient getting medication they should not receive had the patient abstained from eating prior to testing.

An example is cholesterol. A trip at 3 am to get a fast food sandwich could result in a higher cholesterol level that may result in a prescription for medication. It may change that day's glucose level if any medication depends on the numbers in a scale that is referenced for amounts of medication to be administered. Both examples may result in not having accurate readings.

Traveling and Buying Medications Outside the United States

Traveling overseas or outside the United States with medications can be perplexing. The reason why, is prescription medication may not be filled outside the country because of limitations of the provider's licenses to prescribe.

Over the counter medications available in one country may not be purchased in another or may not be offered under the same name. Tylenol is a good example. Tylenol is a pain medication that may be purchased in the United States over the counter. Directions are on the box on how to take it safely. Outside the United States, such as in Mexico or China, Tylenol is called Paracetamol. Thus, if there is time before traveling, checking out what over the counter medications are called. It may be a good idea if there is an emergency.

Another problem is understanding that certain medications or vitamins may not be ready available overseas. Just because a sinus medication or a vitamin is easy to purchase here in the United States does not mean that it will be in the country you are traveling too.

The other problem with over the counter medications available here in the United States may be that the medication may be considered banned or illegal in another country and vice a versa. This can be quite shocking to someone who does not realize they should have been prepared.

The last problem with medication is sticker price shock. Should the medicine in questions be easily located, it may either be very expense or very cheap depending on the country and type of medication. Should the medication be in a pharmacy or apothecary, there will be a specialist who may help in finding a smaller or large amount of desired medication or similar medication that may aid in what is ailing you.

Did you know that Tylenol is not called Tylenol outside the United States of America?

It is called paracetamol.

Traveling with Medicine

Humans are a traveling group of people. Always going somewhere or doing something. What happens when humans need medications while traveling?

Taking enough medication on the trip to cover the days and just a little bit extra in case of a delay, detour, or extended stay.

Take the medication bottles will help with refills should they be needed on a trip. Big pharmacy chains can electronically move prescriptions to another location to be filled if necessary.

Medications may need to be filled in advance or special considerations made when traveling with medication that is needed but may not be allowed in the destination area. This may cause the person to do without the medication or reconsider the travel area.

Is the medication banned or illegal in the country traveling to? Reviewing local laws of the area traveling should be considered if an out of country trip is planned.

How long will the trip last? What happens if there is a delay, extended stay, or rerouting to another country to get to the destination? Will there be enough medication prepared for this to happen?

What would happen if the medication would not be stored properly and would need to be replaced? Is the medication medically necessary for survival and is there a place it could be replaced or a local hospital that may be accessed for treatment?
Is there any special paperwork that needs to accompany the medications? Permission papers, prescription information, and list of medications?

Many things to consider when traveling with medicines but will make the trip pleasant if prepared instead of a nightmare.

Storage of Medications when Traveling

Traveling with medications can be tricky. There are some ways to be prepared.

How long is the trip and will it be in the same country that you are currently in? Traveling locally or in the same country, will allow many people to not need special preparations of storage with medications.

Dry storage of medications will include the original bottles of medications that can be added to bags or suitcases easily. Other options may include daily medication boxes for a few days or weeks storage of medication.

Liquid storage of medications when traveling and going through customs or traveling screenings, may limit liquids to small bottles of 3 ounces. This medication may be sampled or tested to see if it is what the medication says it is to be.

Cold storage is limited to cold packs that last several hours to mini refrigeration's devices. Should the individual be flying and the medication need to be refrigerated, ask the Airlines in advanced for provisions.

Sharps storage is a concern as well. Often the medication delivery system will need the use of a sharp or needle to insert and then dispose of. Many sharps are designed to deliver medication and may be covered or concealed in their device for easily disposable. Those that are not, will need additional arrangements for disposable.

When in doubt about traveling with medications, call the traveling company and speak with a specialist at the pharmacy or apothecary for additional help.

When traveling outside the United States of America, some medications are legal in the United States of America are considered illegal in the destination country and may not be brought into the country. Each country has a list of these medications and should be checked before traveling to avoid any legal problems.

Traveling with a Medicine Bag

Traveling by car frequently may cause a need for a medication bag to arise. Medication bags may contain various things including prescription medications but what else may they contain?

- Over the counter pain medications.
- Nausea and vomiting medications that may need small cups to pour liquid contains into.
- Bandage to cover small to large sores or wounds that could happen.
- Cleaning agents for small to large sores or wounds.
- Ointments for sores, wounds, colds, muscles, and so forth.
- Scissors and a nail file kit.
- Cold or hot packs that may be easily activated.
- Sore or dry throat, cough, and stomach setting medications or drops.
- Eye and ear drops or medications.
- Hand gel cleaner.
- Tissues, paper towels, and moisture towelettes.
- Waste bags for vomit or supplies used.
- A bag to carry it that is easy to access with a lot of pockets but not too big that it cannot be stored easily.

This is a list but may be added or subtracted from for your medicine travel bag. Nice to have on long trips or in emergencies.

Travel Medications and Money

Many times, traveling with medication is necessary. Many health accounts now issue a credit card to pay for medications. This helps keep track of the cost of medications and avoids using travel money for said purchases if needed.

Additional prescription saving cards may allow one to purchase the medications at a discount or free in addition to additional information at the pharmacy or apothecary.

Keeping records of medication use when travel may be considered for a tax write off. Keep good records and consult with your tax adviser.

Other considerations for traveling and money with prescription medications is a digital or paper prescription that may allow for free medication, if the pharmacy or apothecary offers the medication.

Note if there is any need of a medication or prescription paperwork for medication that would need to be presented, such as an insurance card, medication card, identification, and state or government paperwork.

Keep a list of your medications with your travel papers in case of emergency. If traveling to a non-English speaking country, translating the information in to the country's native language may be helpful in an Emergency.

Working on Debt Free with No dryer.

Everyone gets to a point when there is no other item to cut in the budget to get to debt free. Or so I thought, until the dryer broke down a year ago. I have never been one to buy the fancy machines that have lots of bells and whistles.

On average my dryers last about 5-8 years from heavy use. Just could not justify buying something really expensive and my laundry room is not a featured on Pinterest posting boards. My laundry room is a dark part of the basement where the clothes are baptized in saintly soap and water. Clothes are dried, hung up or folded, making their way to a storage space of the person who wears the items.

However, the dryer death of the motor going out, left me with no dryer. To replace with a used refurbish dryer could be a couple hundred. Replacing it with the cheapest new dryer was still a couple hundred.

The problem this time was there was no money. I was trying to downsize the house and the household items. I was trying to cut the debt to give me more freedom. I had put a freeze on buying anything that was deemed unnecessary. Just how necessary is it to own a dryer?

Now the wash machine, was fine. Put clothes in, dump in detergent, and out came clean clothes. Less work than in the pioneering days when cloth was beaten on the rock in the river. A dryer was something I figured I could manage without a few months.

On average, most dryers of four loads of laundry use about 50 cents of electric per load. My electric company includes water in the bill so I will refer to it as just electric. Labor for doing the laundry was not included in this statistic. But figure minimum wage of $8 an hour and labor gets pricey.

It takes my wash machine and dryer to complete a load in 30 to 60 minutes. This is depending on what I put in it. Jeans take longer to dry verses sheets for the bed. Doing a few loads of laundry every day, to keep things done up, is about an hour a day or 7 hours a week. This is about $56 bucks, if you base minimum wage on $8. So $224 a month in labor just to do laundry. Add in the load per hour and that is $3.50 a week or $14 in electric use.

So here was an opportunity to cut the cost. The dryer to purchase and the shipping to get it here and the other one out. The cost of drying items. On average a cheap end dryer, delivery, removal of the old one cost about $500. It can be more or less but let us round up and know there is no sale going on.

One year later, this is what happened. I found that I had completely downsized the wardrobes and needs to wash. A side effect of downsizing and cutting back. I had paired the wardrobe down to two weeks of work attire. One week of winter and one week of summer. A load of whites. A load of towels and/or bedding items.

The rest of the family had also limited their wardrobe to basically dark colors of one load. Gone was the daily washing and now was just key loads of clothes done once a week. This simplify was awe inspiring.

Now here was the catch on the natural drying time. Clothes need so long to dry and the space to dry. Mother Nature could speed up the drying. In the summer of 90-100 degrees days, clothes dried in less than a few hours. In the winter months with lesser heat. It could take clothes to dry up to two days. An extra spin cycle could limit this time but not by much.

The side effects of dry clothes is they aren't the soft and plush of warmth that come out of the dryer. Lint became an issue on some items. Ironing could help with making sure the creases were in the right places instead of the water wicking off the edges look.

What we also noticed was the smell of the clothes. The effort put into the clothes made us more aware of the smell of them. Not just how they looked. Our wardrobe changed out for items that wicked better for drying and dried in shape better. The quality of the clothes became very apparent. Odors did not easy dissolve or were masked by another agent. We changed around the detergents, added more bleach, and even were more aware of where the clothes were dried to prevent leaching of smells into the clothes. I certainly did not appreciate the neighbor mowing the grass when I just hung up my clothes outside.

Items that were not of good quality went to the storage area of do not wear or given away. Suddenly our wardrobes were taking an interesting shape. Our happiness improved. Things were simplified. There was no guessing on what to wear. Choices were paired down. Each day had an outfit. Monday was a blue shirt. Wednesday was a brown shirt. Friday was whatever was left hanging.

Temperature of the day began to take meaning. This is Ohio. Layers are necessary. So what clothes could be layered and still look presentable. Again, the wardrobe took a hit and some items surprised us in the durability of wear.

A year later there is a well-defined look of the wardrobe. Clothing that held up and looks fashionable but not dated. The wash and dry by air helped preserve the items. Occasionally the detergent would not wash out and that would cause rashes on skin. No fun and working with more water in the washer decreased that, as well as, decreasing the soap detergent used.

Eventually, laundry was once a week of about 4-6 loads of items. Hanging things up from the dryer stopped the extra steps involved in a dryer. A lot of planning went into actually doing the laundry. I would have to plan ahead when I could do laundry and the effort of hanging things up inside or outside. Weekends went to realizing the right clothing could be worn over the weekend without adding to the laundry. Eek! Wearing clothes more than once without washing? Barbaric! Until Ohio sent the temperature to freezing and then the comfy warm thermals with one layer over them seemed perfectly just fine. One did become more aware of preventing stains on clothes or wearing good clothing to do work that resulted in need for washing, such as doing yard work or working on the car. Work clothes were changed when arriving home into standard house attire. Things that may have been avoided when a running washer/dryer was the thing.

Financially? 6 loads of laundry per weekend cost $3 in electric and 3 hours of labor of $24. Total of $27 per week or $96 a month. In a year that was $1,152 and just electric was $144 a year.

Fast forward one year later and we purchased a low end fancy dryer. I have spent one weekend washing everything non-stop. Curtains, pillows, blankets, clothes in the house. Surprisingly, I am running out of things mid-Sunday to wash and dry.

The results in the clothes are interesting. The items are not as bright in colors. The lint in the lint trap is amazing and packed full. The clothes come out warm, no wrinkles, and dry quickly. It has been a challenge to keep the washer timed in keeping it flowing. The pause to toss clothes from the washer to the dryer is amusing. Less inspection on if the wash did a good job and more hope the dryer will pick up the slack. Hanging and folding clothes are more reckless as they are already dry. No need to make sure the shoulders dry on the hanger correctly and now more of folding them will help preserve the creases in the folds.

My time with nothing to do has increased. I spend a lot of time trying to be present in the moment. I worried about if the weekend weather was going to be nice to hang out clothes. I was more aware of the cold and heat of the day. I was more attuned to the environment of the day. Weirdly, I am trying to figure out what to do with my time now. Laundry is not a priority as it once was and that is a good thing? Working a full time job and trying to hang out laundry was eating up my time. I felt like I never got a break for rest over the weekend.

Do I feel that I saved money? I feel that I did overall. The electric was cheaper. There was some months that just the basic water cost were charged. Labor increased but my awareness of the environment and time, had me outside more than I normally would have been.

Additionally, my cat would love to run out every Saturday when I hung clothes. He would stay out until the clothes were dry or night fell. Now he's a bit upset over the dryer. His need to guard the clothes is not needed. He has spent the weekend mourning over this loss of activity, laying on the warm clean comforter on the bed.

Will I hang out clothes again? Only if the dryer breaks down. Moving forward I think the dryer will pay for itself in the time I can turn toward other things but the cost of laundry has been based lined for my life style requirements. I can certainly say I did save some money but the side effects of heating the house in the winter, was reflected in the additional heating by other units in the home. Overall, the cutting back of the need to use a dryer was the most cost effective toward going debt free.

Some areas of the United States of America restrict hanging clothes outside. Many countries in the world do not have machines to dry clothes and use hanging racks or other gadgets to meet the needs of drying clothes over night or quickly.

Below the Federal Poverty Level: What Will?

What do you mean a will? I don't have anything. I am poor.
Fact: The United States Federal Poverty level for a single person is income less than $990.00 in 2016.
Fact: That is a total of $11,880 a year in income.
Fact: This is less than $6.185 an hour for full time 40 hours.

Yes, you are poor but this does not mean you cannot have a will. The question is what type of will are we talking about?
There is legal paperwork that everyone should have.

1. A living will. This is a document with an authorizing signature that outlines what a person wants done if they fall sick. Do they want chest compressions done if their heart stops? Do they want medications to be kept comfortable? Do they want to be put on a ventilator?
2. Burial. This may be in the living will, regular will, or just instructions set aside. This includes what type of burial, where the final resting place should be, and if there are any current arrangements set up for this. How to be dressed for final placement, any religious events needed, or another final request.
3. Power of Authority (POA). This is two types of papers. The first POA is for health care and this goes with the living will. This is giving another person permission to speak for you when you cannot and hopefully fill out your wishes. The other type of POA is for assets.
4. A will. This is for the estate and belongs. This will need a POA/executor. This is the person who will handle liquidating the estate and assets.
5. Pets. This may be in the will or directions left behind. Pets with no care or adoptions may be euthanized.
6. Trusts. A trust may be established for any assets. Many States (check with State laws) require assets of over $50,000 to have a living trust or revocable trust. This is when a trust may include the title of the house, car, and collectibles to be later liquidated upon death. This may help prevent delays and probate for the people handling the liquidation of assets. Assets under $50,000 may be consider for a living trust and many not need legal paperwork. Check with state laws for more details. Trust hold advantages for those with deteriorating health conditions and memory problems. Dementia,

Alzheimer's, and Councils on Aging organizations may have more information on how trusts can be beneficial to the individual before and after death.

Thus, every person should have several forms filled out regardless of income. It is not necessary to wait until the deathbed to conduct paperwork. Papers should be done in good health and set aside for when the time comes. Even those who think they are immortal, will have to figure out, who may need to store their belongs one day.

Many legal documents may be found online for free to download and fill out. Always make sure any paperwork competed has been notarize by legal authorities in your State or country, as different laws apply even from State to State. Keep originals in safe locations with copies given to those who may need to have them depending on the situation that may arise. A POA of health care, should have a copy of paperwork and understand what their duties may be if necessary.

Below the Federal Poverty Level: Liquidation of Assets

Fact: The United States Federal Poverty level for a single person is income less than $990.00 in 2016.

Fact: That is a total of $11,880 a year in income.

Fact: Breaking down the $990 and that equates to making $6.185 an hour for full time 40 hours.

A single person reaching the 65-retirement age may find that they did not qualify or pay in enough to get a fat Social Security check. This is reality to many. Many are surprised to find that the fat check is rather skinny and the cost of living are higher than they realized. Many may be taking a hard look at their income and costs without the colored glasses on. It can be shocking.

The choices for this person are slim but not impossible.
Steps to take:

1. File for government help. This is quite hard for many to swallow when they realize they now qualify for things they may have ridiculed others for having. This person many now qualify for money for food. This would-be money that would not come out of the income stream. This will not be a one-time event. This will be ongoing and will have to be updated.
2. Qualify for any social services such as meals on wheels. Meals on wheels offers other things like knowing this person has been checked on when they need to be.
3. Find local pantries and other sources of help in the community that can help. Apply for the resources.
4. Contact the council on aging. There are lots of resources and help weaving the paperwork that is needed to get services in place.
5. Liquidate assets. This may be the hardest thing to do. Assets may not be worth much but anything will help the income base. Other considerations are if taxes are filed, consider donations that may help offset any taxes paid in, lowering the tax bill.

6. Property may need to be sold. This may include vehicles that would cut cost in gas, tags, and insurance costs.
7. Business assets may need to be sold off to supplement living expenses.
8. True retirement. Many business owners want to keep their hands in the work as long as they can. It may be time to decide that this is more of a hobby than a business. Liquidating all the equipment may help fund a bank account to help pay for living conditions.

Here are some ideas for extra income;

- Mowing lawns
- Crossing guards
- Babysitting
- Picking up children from activities
- Collecting scrap, bottles, and cans to recycle
- Making blankets and clothing
- Driving autos to locations for dealers
- Opening or closing stores
- Vacation coverage for homes as sitters or watchers
- Walking dogs
- Helping with city events
- Ushers for museums, opera houses, baseball games
- Helping with concession stands

Below the Federal Poverty Level: How Do You live?

Fact: The United States Federal Poverty level for a single person is income less than $990.00 in 2016.

Fact: That is a total of $11,880 a year in income.

Fact: Breaking down the $990 and that equates to making $6.185 an hour for full time 40 hours.

So how do you live on this type of income? The word living may be subjective. Maslow's Hierarchy of needs are food, water, and shelter.

This means that the single individual must have housing cost low enough that there is money left over to pay for other things. Pew Charitable Trusts in 2014 stated that low income individuals spent approximately 40 percent of their income toward housing/shelter. Thus, approximately about $400 to $500 of the $990 went for housing.

That leaves approximately $500 bucks for everything else. About $100-$125 per week for everything else a person needs. This can quickly be eaten up by a cell phone bill that needs minutes. Food that needs to be cooked/stored and eating out will consume the money very fast with combo meals of $5 per day for one meal. This may be the only meal of the day. Do they qualify for food stamps or do they need to visit pantries for food?

Transportation cost of Uber, cabs, bus, or own vehicles will have to come out of this cost too. Assuming the vehicle is paid off, there is still insurance coverage and gas to get to appointments for health care.

Health care cost may not include everything. Do they fall in the need to pay for medications? Co-pays for insurance? Do they need to qualify for Medicaid?

What about electric? Too hot? Too Cold? Electric bills are not cheap. Is this person even have working heating systems? Is there a working water system? Are they shutting everything off to save money? Are they boiling water so they don't have a water heater eating the electric and keeping the bill high? Are they removing lighting and cutting off all power to keep the bill down? Is this safe or a hazard for them?

Do they have bills that are outstanding and eating into what is left of their money? Do they still owe on things? Do they have credit that needs to be paid monthly? Are they making rash decisions like spending lots of money in risky investments like lotteries and scratch offs hoping for the big payoff that may not come?

What could they do to survive and make it better? It can be quite frightening to find yourself suddenly trying to live on $500 a month.

Income options:

- Paying off a house before working income ends
- Selling off a home after income ends to boost income long term
- Move into an RV or Tiny House to have set expenses and travel or park the home
- Rent out rooms to bring in extra income
- Rent out land for gardens or outside projects
- Rent out garages/basements/attics for storage space
- Sell of autos and use public transportation

Family Expectations

Sometimes families will have expectations. Our family always celebrates on Christmas Eve. Our family always takes the boat out on the lake for Memorial Day. Our family always has the family reunion on the first day of September.

The family learns what the expectations are and will plan for them or not. The problem arises when children become adults and those expectations conflict with each other. The adult children find that they cannot be the same location at the same time. Someone has to give up or change their expectations for the good of the family. This can cause the extended family to become upset because of not being flexible. It can also cause misery on the family that are trying to meet everyone's needs, including their own needs.

Families that learn to be flexible will become happier than those who refuse to budge. Yet, some family events may swallow in other families with their traditions and events and learn to grow happily.

Planning for the year will help many family members. Some families change their traditions and start new ones. Instead of everyone gathering for winter holidays, they exchange the time for a vacation everyone can go on. This helps those family members who work during the holiday, to still get to be part of the holiday event.

Families may even grow to include "adopted" family members. Many families find they enjoy the same types of fun and events and plan to holiday together. Other families may decide that individual or smaller family events work better for them.

Outlining the holiday events with families can help prevent a lot of sadness and upset when the holidays return each year.

Family Money

Money is always a topic with families. There needs to be an income of money resources that takes care of the family needs. The family needs to decide how many members will supply and access the resources. What the resources should be used towards and if any of the resources should be applied to items, care, or savings for the future family needs.

Children may or not have access to the resources. Access may be in allowances, money earned for chores or grades, and holiday events.

Adult members may decide on a financial plan and how the resources will be applied. Members may decide on all or portions of income going to different family needs or individual needs.

Planning will need to include money for emergencies. Some emergencies funds may be for when the washer or dryer quits, possible hurricane evacuation, or there is an accident or illness. Each emergency fund will be dependent upon the family and their possible needs.

Money funds may need to be set up for during live expectations, such as child care or adult care. Funds may need to be set up for the passing of a family member. Families may know that a member's life will be ending and may prepare for the events to follow. This is when families will need to consider what type of paperwork may be needed to be in place for a family member. The paperwork may need to cover guardianship for care of children and funding for future education. Paperwork regarding how assets will be distributed and when may need to be listed in a trust or additional paperwork that will need to be addressed by lawyers and court systems.

Families may go through a difficult time with money. This is when things happen beyond the families control and preparedness. Funds or income may drop to zero. Families may have to reach out to outside resources to meet the living needs. This may include relocating or dividing up the family to meet the needs. Families with financial trouble may need to reach out to counseling for emotional and financial help.

Families who see money as a tool to achieving the life style and meeting their needs may find the family is happier than those who do not use this idea.

Family Pets

Family members may decide they wish to have a pet. This decision can be easy or quite an obstacle. The idea to accept a pet into the family may be spontaneous, planned, temporary, or a life changing event.

Pets come in all shapes, types, and needs. Goldfish won at the Fair verses taking over care of a pet of a deployed military family member, will have different needs and expectations. The family will need to make sure all members understand the care needs for the pet and the expectations of each family member with the pet.

Most animal's needs are simple; food, water, love, a place to sleep, and cleanup of body fluids.

The cost of feeding a cat verses a horse will need to be added into the family budget. The budget may or not cover the expenses of having a family pet. If the budget changes and the cost is no longer possible, this may lead to the family needing to "rehome" the animal or take it to a shelter to be "rehome" or "put down". Such events may happen when an elder of the family passes on and the pet needs to be adopted, rehome, or euthanized.

Pets with wealthy owners may have paperwork in place that will take care of their needs. Family will need to know where the paperwork is and the legal ramifications of not following through with these types of legal contracts and papers.

The pet may not work out. Sometimes the pet has a short life and the family members may new to the grieving processes and burial ideas. These are valuable learning experiences to the young and teaches coping skills for later in life. Grieving by a family member that continues on for months, the family member may need to seek counseling.

Replacing a pet. Sometimes pets pass on or "cross the rainbow bridge". The loss of the missing pet may be too great in the family and the family may consider getting a new pet. Not so much to replace the pet but to continue to provide and outlet for the love the family wishes to express in caring.

Each family will need to decide if a pet's needs can be met and if that is a good decision for the family. Sometimes a pet's needs cannot be met and the family will decided not to have a pet.

Family Meetings

There will be times when families will need to get together and meet over serious things. Family meetings may be simple and covering over new changes in the household like adding new rules or demonstrations on how to do new chores. The meetings may include visuals of charts, video, and paperwork the will need to be implemented. Meetings may be short or scheduled for several hours to cover more serious content or involve speakers, such as lawyers, providers, or clergy.

New families may organize meetings to be short, over simple problems with solutions, and implementation of those ideas. Those ideas may include introducing a chore chart with rewards, planning a vacation, or how to properly take care of a new pet.

Establish families may meet once a week or month to share problems and solutions in caring for elder family members and updates on what the provider of care has said regarding the family member. This is the time when discussions of important papers may be discussed.

Merging families may meet periodically to arrange holiday events and child care events to keep things moving smoothly for everyone.

Extended families may meet to organize the family reunion, collection and storage of family heirlooms and heritage items, and details of family history to be arranged to pass on.

Family emergencies may need to activate the implementation of a telephone tree of communication or update social media to alert family of events unfolding that need emergency actions.

Every family will need to decide how a family meeting may be helpful to organizing and keep their family functioning over time. Some families may not need to meet but once in a while and other families will need mandatory meets to keep events moving forward.

Family Quality Over Quantity Tips

There will come a time in every family member's life that the quantity of time is more important than quality of time. This is when the family needs to keep things simple, enjoyable, and memorable.

Saying hello and goodbye. Having a traditional greeting, phrase of words, and important terms that are endearing to the person saying it or receiving it in the exchange.

Keeping events simple. Some families will want to keep the events the same year after year. This may be acceptable but the time will come when the family changes and the events will be too heartbreaking to continue the same way.

New traditions. Do not be afraid to start them. Sometimes traditions start because of sad event turned happy. It is okay to mix it up or add fun.

Take the time to speak to everyone at each event for a few minutes.

Be an active listener during the time you are spending with the family member. If you are not familiar with what they are discussing, ask questions and give them a chance to explain it to you.

Advice works better when it is requested than absently given out like candy. When giving advice, keep it factual and geared to be helpful in decision making, instead of authoritarian and that is the way it is.

Mamasan's Water Park

When the children were little, I took all their outside toys and put them on a tarp surrounded a water sprinkler. I turned it on and the water turned the toys into a water park of fun. They loved it. I would then leave them in the care of their Father and I would leave for work. As adults they remember Mamasan's water park. They don't remember a teary eyed Mother leaving for 12 hour night shift, who only got to spend 5 minutes with them before she left. They only remember the moment of fun and not how long they played or how long I spent with them. Create memory moments.

Pre-Existing Condition

What does it mean to have a pre-existing condition? It means you were born or acquired a condition that may need ongoing treatment throughout your life.

Why is this important with insurance companies? This is important with insurance companies because of what they consider a pre-existing condition means, it may cost more to pay the bills to keep the individual healthy. To the insurance company, pre-existing means they can keep customers or turn them away because they do not see any money or profit in keep the customers.

The insurance company may lack the ability to contract with suppliers, pharmaceutical companies, hospitals, and providers to keep cost low to keep profit high for the insurance company. The insurance companies may lose money on an individual because of a condition.

Example:
An individual pays the insurance company $500 a month to have insurance. That is $6,000 a year. If the individual sees their provider for blood pressure or hypertension problems, the patient will need medication to keep it in the normal range and stay healthy.

The individual sees the provider every three months and gets their medication with no other problems. The provider charges the insurance company $200 per visit. The insurance company may or not pay the full amount. The year of visits will be $800. The insurance company has made $5,200 profit.

The pharmacy will charge $4 for the one month of medications. $4 x 12 months = $48 charged to insurance and minus the $5,200, the profit is $5,152 to the insurance company.

Now the insurance company may decide there should be some skin in the game for the individual and may decide they need to pay a co-payment. The co-payment is due at the visit and can range from $5 to $50+ per visit. This is money the individual pays including the monthly amount. This means the insurance company will still need to pay as well but minus the copay and the insurance company keeps more of the monthly money.

The insurance company may decide a high deductible before they pay. Thus, the individual pays ALL the deductible before the insurance pays anything. This may be with or without a co-pay. This means that if an individual has $5,000 deductible, all that money must be paid. When the provider charges the insurance company, the insurance will pay zero. The bill then goes to the patient to pay all the bill. The amount is then minus the deductible. If the patient has enough bills that go over the $5,000 then the insurance begins to pay.

As you can see, the patient is paying a monthly cost of $500 to have insurance but it will not even pay any bills until the deductible is paid first. So, if you do not have over $5,000 in annual bills the insurance is not worth anything. The true cost is really $500 monthly payment and $417 a month or $917 a month for insurance that will not pay anyone but the insurance company.

The individual will need to still pay the provider and the pharmacy for their medications.

When purchasing insurance or obtaining insurance through an employer, always review all the fine print. Make sure you understand what you are purchasing and what it covers. Do know if an insurance covers 80%, the 20% owed may be due at the time of service. This is in addition to any copays or deductibles.

When purchasing insurance, be sure to find out what medications will or will not be covered. Many patients are surprised to find out that medications are very expensive. Especially medications advertised on television.

Do know many pharmacies have 4-5 dollar list of many common medications that will help when insurances will not cover medications.

What Happens with Pre-Existing Conditions

What is a pre-existing condition? It means you were born or acquired a condition that may need ongoing treatment throughout your life.

What happens when you have a pre-existing condition and get sick? With all pre-existing conditions, there may be the need to see a provider or seek hospital treatments. This means that the patient will need to make regular visits to see a provider for health care problems and get medications and so forth.

Anything can be a pre-existing condition that causes an individual to need care ongoing.

There is no problem with the patient getting the care they need. The problem begins when the individual has no way to provide payment for the visits. There are many ways that a patient can pay for visits.

Cash. The individual can pay the entire bill with cash, check, or credit cards. The problem begins when the cost of care becomes too great of a cost.

This is when individuals seek out insurances. Sometimes companies provide insurance for their employees. The employee may or not have to pay monthly amounts out of their check at a discounted rate given by the insurance company to the company, who is offering the insurance to the employee.

This may mean the employee will need to pay a co-payment at the time of the visit. This is the agreed amount of money the employee has agreed to pay and the insurance will pick up the rest of the bill. This is in addition to the cost of the monthly amount.

The other option is a Medicaid. This insurance may pay for the entire amount of the visit and no payments to the individual. The problem here is when the individual does not keep the paperwork up to date or no longer eligible for the insurance. Then the individual needs to pay the entire amount at the visit if the eligibility is no longer in place. Medicaid is money that the State of the individual's residence provides to the individual for health care. States that have increased their Medicaid coverage do so with funds provided from Federal help. If the Federal help declines, then the States may limit the coverage or the items covered under insurance.

A pre-existing condition can be seen by a provider, the problem is the person with the pre-existing condition affording the care with limited resources.

Pre-existing conditions;

- Pregnancy
- Birth defects
- Surgeries
- Chronic health histories
- Smoking
- Alcohol consumption
- Body Mass Indexes (BMI) not in normal limits
- And more...

Deductibles for Insurances

Why do insurances have deductibles? The insurance company decides that the patient needs to have "skin in the game" and will ask for a deductible. This means that there is a set amount of money that must be paid before the insurance will be begin paying.

This is for all insurances. A deductible may allow the insurance company to provide insurance with lower monthly payments. To get a monthly payment to have coverage from the insurance company, the deducible will be higher than the regular rate.

Example:
To have car insurance for $125 a month, the deductible is $1,000. This means that the monthly bill to the insurance company is $125. If the car is in an accident and needs to be fixed, the individual must pay $1,000 first. The money may go to the insurance company or is directed to the place fixing the car as part of the payment agreed will fix the car as good as new again.

To have health insurance payments at $500 a month, the deductible is $5,000. This means that the individual pays $500 a month to the insurance company. This is regardless if the person sees a provider for any health care problems or emergencies. When the individual does see a provider, the cost of the visit is paid by the individual as part of the deductible. The insurance will pay zero or not "kick in" until the full $5,000 has been paid.

Agreeing on a high or lower deductible is up to the individual. This will help them to keep or not keep coverage for insurance.

This happens regardless if there is a pre-existing health problem or not. A pre-existing health problem may result in the insurance company seeing no profit in providing insurance and deny the individual. Thus, the individual may be able to pay monthly and the deductible but may not have enough money to pay an entire hospital bill. This is when the insurance would be helpful in this situation.

Pre-Existing Payment Options

What are ways to pay for a pre-existing condition?

A pre-existing condition means there is a health problem that is ongoing for the individual. This means the individual needs to seek out health care on a regular basis to stay within their considerations of healthy and functioning.

Each pre-existing health problem has limitations on how well or healthy the individual is.

If a person does not have a pre-existing health problem, the person is considered "healthy". Payments to remain healthy, may be very low in cost.

A person with low health care cost may be able to pay in cash, check, or credit card.

A person with high levels of health care needs may need to inquire into insurance to help offset the high amounts of payments with insurance. This is when the individual agrees to pay co-payments, deductibles, and monthly fees to keep insurance to help pay over the amount of health care needs throughout the year. This is helpful when health care cost is over thousands of dollars a month in provider care, treatments, and medications needed to maintain a "healthy" lifestyle.

Health plans or concierge care. This is when the individual acts as their own company or buys into a plan provided by a health care or company. This is a set rate cost for care per visit or monthly payments over time for a future visit(s) for care.

The Question of "How Hard Can It Be?"

How hard can it be, is often the question we briefly ask ourselves when we attempt a task in life. How hard can be discerned by how much experience an individual had in the past with a task.

Example:
First grade. There were preparations that were made for this grade. The need to know the first grader's name, address, contact information, and basic skills such as alphabet and counting to a set number correctly needs to be accomplished.

Now how hard comes into play when the first grader never was exposed to any other schooling prior to this event. No pre-school or Kindergarten and the child will be experiencing everything new for the first time. First time leaving family to go to school, trying and learning to make friends, and trying to figure it all out. This may cause a lot of emotional and lessons burnt into the mind on how coping skills were earned through learning. Coping skills may result in helping the child deal and cope with future experiences. A bad experience and the child may shy away. A good experience and the child will try more experiences.

How hard may be easier for those who have attended some form of educational system and the child may already excel in many of the task to be taught at the first-grade level due to years of prior experience. The child may know how to even read and write. The child knows how to push to get to the chair, get in line fast, and already understands the outcomes of why or why not things are happening. The child has no qualms leaving the family, behavior may be more conditioned to set environment, and the child may have developed quite a few coping skills by this point.

This does not mean that the child who was prepared early will succeed more later, it just gives the child more resources of experiences to pull from verses the child who did not receive the prepared education but may have been expose to other experiences of equal or greater value for life preparation. Children not attending school early may have more adult skills due to spending time and building relationships with adults, instead of children.

From this example, we have discerned that prior education or experiences may reduce the "how hard is it?" question. This can also keep a lot of folks from trying new things because they are comfortable with their frame of education and experiences. This can cause happiness for many and will relate into stress when forced out of their scope of education and experiences when trying or forced into new experiences.

Thus, one with a lot of experiences in various types of skills may see the hard part not as hard as an individual with no experiences. No experience person may even think such a skill, job, event, or activity is out of their reach to even attempt. This does not mean they shouldn't attempt it. It just means it may simply be harder than they thought when it is done. The coping skills they have learned will help them as they move through the task to either failure or success and at this point it becomes very subjective answer to the question of "how hard could it be?"

Coping skills are created when children are allowed to play alone and with other children. As children grow, encouraging to explore, play, and learn with guidance helps coping skills to form. Trying new foods, adventures, and learning about people help form experiences to learn from and use as they grow into adults. Adults can help form coping skills by understanding they are responsible for their feeling and how they react to others. Understanding that constant failures creates success as children and adults find ways to make things work out.

Set Meals for Weight Loss

A patient is already eating health meals and may have limited their meals to two a day, may still be trying to figure out how they are not losing any weight? Where else can they cut out calories? It can be truly frustrating.

What are they putting into their mouths when they leave are not eating meals? Many do not realize that the snacking is where the calories are slipping in. A bit here, a cookie there, a handful of this or that and they move on. Perhaps a quick check to see if the refrigerator light is still on may lead to grabbing a bite of something in it and moving on to something else.

Snacking is the term for this but good marketing and advertisement has us believing that snacking is opening up a bag of chips, candy, or a quick prepackage power bar to get through the day is necessary. True, a prepackaged power bar might be a quick substitute for a business person on the go missing lunch because a meeting ran over or a Mom dropping off kids and picking up elder parents to take to a provider appointment that runs through lunch.

Snacks average from 100 to 250 calories per package or handful. Now it takes approximately 250 calories removed from a diet per day to lose one pound a week. If you are eating between meals, this may be where your calories for gaining weight are really coming from and not your two meals a day.
How do you overcome this problem? Set meal times.

Example:
Non-breakfast folks (no morning meal will eat approximately 10 am to 2 pm for their first meal. Their second meal will be approximately 8 hours later, around at 6pm to 10 pm at night. As you can see there is a lot of room for snacking here. Snacking mid-day, afternoon, and late evening. Lots of places to sneak in calories.

Breakfast folks will pick either lunch or dinner as their second meal. This means that early morning from 5am to 8 am and then around 5pm to about 8pm. That's a long time for the body to try and keep the energy levels. Again, sneaking in a bite mid-day, afternoon, and then later after meals may happen.

How to get around the snacking? The body needs to keep the energy levels up. The body converts calories into sugar. Much like a car uses gas to run. No gas and the car goes nowhere. Same with the body. The energy levels tank and the body begins sending messages to do something to raise the levels again. This is when snacking happens.

So instead of snacking, add in the third meal at a set time. The average human will stay awake approximately 12-16 hours per day. Divide this up equally and the three meals will be 4 to 6 hours apart throughout the day. Breakfast would be upon waking or shortly after waking. This begins the next 4-6 hours until the next meal, followed by another 4-6 hours for the next meal.

Breakfast is at 8 am. Lunch is at 12-2 pm. Supper is at 4-6 pm. This would mean no late-night snacking and bedtime would be 8pm for a 12-hour day and midnight for a 16-hour day for those up at 8am.

Try three set meal times to avoid snacking for weight loss.

Normal weight loss a week should be 1-2 pounds.

Normal weight loss for a month should be 4-8 pounds.

Normal weight loss for 3 months should be 12-32 pounds.

Normal weight loss for 6 months should be 24-48 pounds.

Normal weight loss for 12 months should be 52-104 pounds.

Understand that this is estimated weight loss and subject to each individual's efforts and circumstances.

Understand that weight loss claims of a lot of weight lost in one to two weeks may really be dehydration or evacuation of GI tract. When the body re-hydrates or the GI tract fills up with food/waste again, the weight will return.

Do not limit calories under 1,000 calories per day. This will cause the body to believe it is starving and weight loss may be halted as the body becomes a "hoarder" and will hang on to food.

Weight Loss Games

Like many partners or married patients, both will be overweight and both will need to lose weight. Here is an advantage for many. A weight loss partner that shares in the same bad or good habits. So, when motivation is lacking with one partner, the other partner may benefit from getting encourage to go for a walk or push the plate back at meals.

Most folks do love games and instead of competing against each other to see who can lose the most weight, view the goal as a combined team effort.

Example:
Team Goins. Female Goins weighted in at 244 and Male Goins weighted in at 271. This is a combined total weight of 515 pounds to lose.

The goal is to lose one pound a week each but all weight loss is a combined effort for the team. Meaning, taking a cookie for the team isn't going to help the team lose weight.

It is important to keep with the same scale and same items or clothes or a dry naked weight at the same time of day per week. The reason is that the results can be skewed.

Team Goins weights in weekly and Female Goins lost 4 pounds. She has met her goals and added 3 pounds for Team Goins. Male Goins lost 8 pounds. He has met his goal of one pound lost and added 7 pounds for Team Goins. Team Goins is already winning with a team effort of 12 pounds lost from the 515 total to the new total of 503. Go Team Goins!

As you can see. Each team member has met their goals and team goals too. While it is great to say, I lost one pound or four pounds, it is going to be way much cooler to say Team Goins lost 12 pounds already! Motivation goes up and working for the team's effort benefits both team members. If one team member gets side tracked, the team still may lose weight and help re-direct struggling team members to stay positive and with goals because they are still winning at the weight loss game.

Another fun way to enjoy weight loss is to compare what your loss of weight might be.

- 10# = medium bowling ball
- 20# = Automobile tire
- 30# = A microwave
- 40# = A border collie dog
- 50# = A bale of hay
- 60# = A punching bag
  And so forth...

Weight Loss and Where to Start

Patients will tell me that they are already eating two meals a day or eating healthy. Where else can they cut out calories? Looking past, the healthy meals and calorie intake of those meals, you need to see what else isn't a meal that is causing calorie intake.

Beverages is one place that calories sneak in. Why Lisa, I am only drinking one cup of coffee. How big is this cup of coffee? Is it 12, 36, 48 ounces per sitting? Are you drinking it half way down and refilling to warm it up and not realizing you are drinking more than 12 ounces but really 16 ounces? How much extra sugar and creamer have been added?

I have seen folks purchase a morning coffee to drink for breakfast and to sip on all day. I have watched them add sugars to their coffees. Example here is real sugar is 16 calories a packet. It takes 3 packets to flavor the coffee to taste in and 8-ounce cup. That is 48 calories of sugar total. Now let us multiply the size of the cup and sugar. A 16-ounce cup of coffee includes 6 packets of sugar and equal to 96 calories. A 32-ounce cup is 512 calories and for those super coffee lovers and 48 ounces is six cups of coffee is a whopping 2,304 calories. If you are finishing off the pot of coffee at work or home, a pot of coffee is approximately 8 cups or 64 ounces of coffee. The sugar added at three packets to each cup of coffee in the pot? This is an astounding total of 3,072 calories of liquid with sugar. We didn't even add in the calories for milk or flavored creamer. That is 1,072 calories over a 2000 calorie recommended diet.

Now it takes on average 250 calories a day to lose one pound a week. Looking at 2,304 calories that is approximately a 12-pound weight loss in just liquid calories per week!

Measurements:

1 Jigger = 1.5 US fluid ounces

1 US teaspoon = 0.67 US fluid ounces

1 cup = 8.12 US fluid ounces

1 US Pint = 16 US fluid ounces

1 liter = 33.82 US fluid ounces

1 US liquid gallon = 128 US fluid ounces

Losing Weight Goals

Patients often have no idea how to lose weight or where to even start. Many have a Body Mass Index (BMI) that classifies them as obese. So just losing a few pounds will go un-noticed by anyone around and that makes the motivation even harder.

Realistically, what can a person do? Simplify the goal is one way. Often, a person with a BMI has a lot of weight to lose. It can be overwhelming to them. It seems like an impossible idea. First thing to realize that often we are talking about more than 25 pounds to lose, we are talking closer to 50 pounds with higher BMIs.

Setting a goal. The goal will be to lose one pound a week. Now this may or not sound exciting to someone who is very overweight. They may want to lose the weight quick or be dis-illusion that losing weight is even possible.

Losing one pound a week is equal to 4 pounds a month. In 12 weeks, that is equal to 12 pounds for a short-term goal. Short term goals are ways to begin working on the weight loss. Patients can return to the provider and see that they are indeed, successful at losing weight.

Long term goals will be one pound a week for 52 weeks. This will result in 52 pounds in their weight loss. This means that approximate calories to be removed from the diet is 250 calories. More aggressive patients may want to step the goal up to 2 pounds for 52 weeks and this will result in 104 pounds lost. This would mean that 500 calories a day would need to be removed daily from the caloric intake. To a very obese person tipping the scales over 300 pounds, this would be a lot of success to them with 104 pounds in their weight loss.

Patients who have high BMIs may benefit from regular weight ins with their provider to help keep motivation up and weight loss increased.

BMI under 18 is considered under weight

BMI 18-25 is considered normal

BMI over 25 is considered over weight

BMI over 30 is considered obese.

Realistic Weight Loss Goals

It is beyond miserable to tell someone who is obese that they need to lose weight. Often, the weight loss needed is 50 to 100 pounds or more. The demand by society that this happens quickly can be heart wrenching to the individual.

The realistic weight loss goal is one pound a week. Now this may not seem like a lot to the individual and may not be as quick as they would wish but it is fast enough when you think in long term goals.

First, the life span is not going to change. Time is going to flow regardless if the person is losing weight or not. A year is going to go by no matter what the person eats or not. Thus, if the individual losses one pound a week, in 52 weeks, the person is going to lose 52 pounds. If the weight goal is 2 pounds a week, this is 104 pounds. That is significant weight loss!

A person can look completely different in one year or 52 weeks by losing only one to two pounds a week.

Why is this so awesome? Mentally, it is an easy task to focus on. One pound a week is only struggling with 7 days to lose one pound. Short term goals that are easy to achieve every week. It keeps the individual from being overwhelmed and quit trying. Losing 100 pounds is overwhelming but to think about it as 2 pounds for 52 weeks is 104 pounds and over the goal set. The individual just needs to understand that the weight loss is going to take time and results will not be noticed by everyday company until the weight loss has been significant. This can be frustrating to rely on compliments from others. Do not let this stop the goals for weight loss.

It only takes approximately 250 calories eliminated from the diet to lose one pound a week. Keeping up the 250 calories eliminated from the diet will keep the individual losing weight. This may be as easy as giving up two cans of pop/soda or one candy bar a day.

In summary, the short-term goal is one to two pounds a week. The long-term goal is one to two pounds a week for 52 weeks or a year. This is doable goals.

Eliminating 250 calories every day for one week is 1,750 calories per week.

Eliminating 500 calories every day for one week is 3,500 calories per week.

The average number of calories in a hamburger or hotdog bun is 120 calories.

The average number of calories in commercially prepared white bread is 80 calories per slice or 160 calories per two slices.

The average medium size French fires have 365 calories.

Losing Weight with Magnesium Supplements

Are you experiencing muscle cramps? Do you shake at night before you follow asleep? Are your legs restless and shake at night? Do you crave chocolate? Do you eat chocolate by the bags not the bars?

Then, the individual may have a magnesium deficiency. All the symptoms mention relates to lack of magnesium in the body. Lack of magnesium can cause the body to cramp, shake before falling asleep, legs to shake, and chocolate to be consumed as meals instead of treats.

Health care providers may draw blood levels to discern if magnesium is low in the body. If the levels are low, insurances may pay for prescription magnesium.

Other options are to purchase magnesium over the counter. Should there be concerns or questions of the choices available, consult a pharmacist where purchasing magnesium to meet the individual's needs.

Individuals craving chocolate will notice that their cravings will diminish resulting in weight loss. On average a chocolate candy bar is 250 calories. If the individual is eating one candy bar a day, then stopping, will result in one pound a week loss with replacement of magnesium in a supplement.

Know the difference

Magnesium **citrate** is used as a laxative as it increases water in the intestines.

Magnesium **oxide** may help with night muscle cramps in legs at night.

Needing Supplements to Help with Weight Loss

Many individuals try to lose weight but have a budget that isn't helpful in reaching the needed vitamin and mineral content. This is when taking a daily supplemental multivitamin is helpful. A multivitamin will help the individual get the daily requirements needed when the nutrition level of available food is not present. If a person is eating less than three meals a day, the individual may need a multivitamin supplement.

Basic multivitamins are fine for use. Many with insurances will find that if their provider prescribes them, the insurances will pay for a generic version.
The vitamin will be eliminated in urine daily and it is important to drink the norm of 64 ounces of water per day. A good gauge to follow, is the urine should be clear when eliminated to know if enough water has been ingested.

Vitamins are a combination of water and fat soluble. This means that some of the vitamins need to be replaced daily, such as vitamin B's and C's and other vitamins like vitamin D3 builds up in the body. This can translate into the individual taking vitamins for 30 days or a month before they may notice any difference. Individuals with low levels of vitamins may notice quicker results in how they feel.

Always take a vitamin with several bites of food in the am hours of the individual's morning schedule. Vitamins love to go to work when they reach the stomach and the adverse effects may make the individual have slight gastric upset if not taken with food.

Vitamins break down into two basic categories.

Water soluble vitamins do **not** build up in the body and are flushed out of the body.

Fat soluble vitamins do build up in the body and may result in toxic levels if not managed correctly.

Realistic weight loss goals

It is beyond miserable to tell someone who is obese that they need to lose weight. Often, the weight loss needed is 50 to 100 pounds or more. The demand by society that this happens quickly can be heart wrenching to the individual.

The realistic weight loss goal is one pound a week. Now this may not seem like a lot to the individual and may not be as quick as they would wish but it is fast enough when you think in long term goals.

First, the life span is not going to change. Time is going to flow regardless if the person is losing weight or not. A year is going to go by no matter what the person eats or not. Thus, if the individual losses one pound a week, in 52 weeks, the person is going to lose 52 pounds. If the weight goal is 2 pounds a week, this is 104 pounds. That is significant weight loss!

A person can look completely different in one year or 52 weeks by losing only one to two pounds a week.

Why is this so awesome? Mentally, it is an easy task to focus on. One pound a week is only struggling with 7 days to lose one pound. Short term goals that are easy to achieve every week. It keeps the individual from being overwhelmed and quit trying. Losing 100 pounds is overwhelming but to think about it as 2 pounds for 52 weeks is 104 pounds and over the goal set. The individual just needs to understand that the weight loss is going to take time and results will not be noticed by everyday company until the weight loss has been significant. This can be frustrating to rely on compliments from others. Do not let this stop the goals for weight loss.

It only takes approximately 250 calories eliminated from the diet to lose one pound a week. Keeping up the 250 calories eliminated from the diet will keep the individual losing weight. This may be as easy as giving up two cans of pop/soda or one candy bar a day.

In summary, the short-term goal is one to two pounds a week. The long-term goal is one to two pounds a week for 52 weeks or a year. This is doable goals.

Losing Weight by Drinking Water.

Do you even drink water? Most folks drink some water but then drink other drinks through the day instead of water. Water rehydrates the body and will help the mind be more alert, the skin look cleaner, and help with gastrointestinal problems by balancing out the ph.

The recommendation is that 8 ounce glasses is the serving size. The individual needs to drink 8 glasses. This is a total of 64 ounces of water a day. That translates into the body needing half a gallon of water per day on average.

Now 8 glasses of water may seem like a lot but when you spread it out throughout 24 hours, and individual would only be drinking one glass every 3 hours. Realistically, many individuals are awake 12-16 hours per day. Again, one glass of water every hour would not be a difficult task to accomplish.

But what if you are already drinking the "normal" amount of water? Then, the goal would be increasing it to one gallon of water a day or 16 glasses that measure 8 ounces. Now this would translate into one glass every 16 hours or increasing the glass size to consume more in less time. Typically, most serving sizes can be 12, 16, 24, 36, and 64 ounces in cup sizes.

Now one might think that is a lot of water but pop/soda is sold in these sizes and consumed in one sitting with a meal. What if the pop/soda was changed out for water? On average, this would be 100 calories not consumed in 8 ounces. It takes 250 calories eliminated to lose one pound a diet. So, 8 ounces x 100 calories equaling 800 calories not consumed on average. Plenty of a difference to see the results on a scale by just drinking water instead of pop/soda.

Try drinking only water to lose weight. Maybe it is all you need to do.

Pay attention to the ounces verses milliliters in water bottles.

16.9 ounces will translate into 500 milliliters of water. If you are counting water bottles in 16 ounces and drink 8 bottles of water a day. Don't forget to add the 0.9 fluid x 8 bottles = 7.2 ounces per day.

Losing Weight with a Nutrition App

A lot of patients have no idea how to lose weight or even where to start. This is when starting with a nutrition app on a cell phone is helpful. Download the application to the cell phone and then begin a log of all the food eaten per day. This can show the person just where their trouble spots are in their diets or lifestyle of eating.

The nutrition apps will break the food down into carbohydrates, fats and proteins. This help the individual target in more on what maybe causing the weight gains. It can show if there is too much to too little of carbohydrates, fats and proteins. By watching the data, the individual can then adjust eating intake to balance out the outcomes desired.

Other advantages of nutrition apps are seeing where too much salt or sodium is hidden in the daily log of food ingested. It will also show mineral and vitamin content. Helpful for those with anemias and electrolyte balance issues.

If you are struggling to figure out what is wrong in your diet, consider a free downloadable nutrition app on your cell phone.

A weight app of interest for cell phones or computers is

www.myfitnesspal.com

This app is free for the basic form and allows the user to log in food, water, exercise, and keep track of calories. It can also break down the intake of food into fats, carbohydrates, and proteins.

Definitions:

Carbohydrates: are sugars (complex and simple) that break down into in the body into glucose.

Fats: are saturated and unsaturated fatty acids.

Proteins: are made up of amino acids.

Our body made up of 42% protein or 15% the mass of the average person.

Diet Failure and Calorie Counting

What is calorie counting? Calories are divided up into fats, carbohydrates, and proteins.

Each type creates a calorie that takes x effort to remove it from the body or create weight in the body.

Like any rich person given extra money, they may store it or spend it. The body will do the same thing with calories.

The average body needs about 2000 calories a day. Some bodies will need more or less depending on the function or disease process that is invading the body. The calories are a combination of the three types. If weight gain is needed, then more carbohydrates are needed in the body mix of calories. If weight loss is required, then less carbohydrates and fats should be ingested and more proteins should be required in the mix.

The incorrect mix of calories will also result in the wrong or desire effects. Too many carbohydrates will result in busting
down into simple sugars and could have the wrong results if the person is a diabetic. This could increase the blood sugars in the body.

A mix of low carbohydrates and increased proteins may help the body to shed weight or build up desire muscle mass. Fats may help the person to feel full without over eating in the carbohydrate section of foods.

Once a person begins counting calories, be sure the mix of calories is the desired type for weight loss/gain or to prevent disease effects.

Note:

The Federal Government estimates that the average American consumes 2,000 calories per day in their diet. All food on nutritional labels are based on 2,000 calories. This may need to be adjusted if the person is not eating a 2,000 calories per day. This may be why a diet may fail.

Diet Failure and Sleep

One of the fails with dieting is not getting enough sleep. Many dieters over look this key success for losing weight. On average the human can be up 12 to 16 hours per day. This means the other time is in sleep mood of 8 to 12 hours. Many artificially keep awake with beverages of caffeine and sugar. This can destroy dieting attempts really fast.

Sugar is instant burn calories for the body and can cause weight gain.
Caffeine can cause artificial awakeness and begin causing the body to function artificially.
Insomnia prevents the body from re-booting into a natural mode that allows functions to move naturally.

Sadly, the body is not at internet speed and many humans are not cool with this. The expectations are then artificially heightened with drinks and medications. Eventually, the body just cannot keep up regardless of the additives.

The underestimated sleeping of 8 to 12 hours can refresh the body faster and quicker than many additives can hyper-jump it.
Poorly depleted bodies, forced into the slavery of insomnia to function, will eventually begin shutting down systems.
Immunity will crash and the body will become sick. Once the body is sick, it will take more than just additives to make it
better. It will take sleep to reset the body. If the body is so depleted, it may take several weeks of regular routine sleeping
to rebound the body.

Therefore, do not just look at your additives, calories, but the amount of sleep per day. Increasing sleep may help weight
loss goals to be achieved a lot quicker.

> The 8 hour sleep schedule was designed when Ford Automobile Company began the factory line. This began the 3 shifts per day of 8 hours. Before this time frame, the general public did not sleep 8 hours at night. It was normal to wake up after several hours to attend to the fire in the hearth, watch through the night, and check on the animals.

Diet Failure and Stopping It

Is the diet short term or life changing. This is the big problem with diet failure. You are either in or you are not. Just like many TV shows that show massive weight loss and then those participants gain it back when the diet is not followed any more.
There is the need to know that all diets will fail when the individual does not realize this is forever changes.

Yes, diets can be short term or long term. Many short term diets are to get bodies back into the condition they were in before
the diet.

Short Term Examples:
Losing weight after having an infant. Often the woman was at the desired weight before the birth of the child and wishes to remove the added weight gained for a successful pregnancy.

Diets may often have desire effects, such as preparing for an event or enlistment. The person may need to lose or gain weight before this type of event happens to be successful.

Long Term Examples:
Losing or gaining weight to keep the body at a required or desired weight. This will require the individual to keep the same
type of exercise and food intake regular forever. Not everyone realizes that to keep a body at a desire weight, this can mean
keeping same routine of food over and over. It may result in never eating certain foods ever again. This is not always something many can continue to do to keep the desire effect and this results in diet failure.

Ways to prevent diet failure? Cheat day. One day per month or months, where the person may cheat by eating foods they have restricted from the diet to maintain the body. Often, a cheat day is after a big event and used to celebrate. Once the day is over, the individual returns to the regular diet. Many find that after restricting x food from their diet, that when a cheat day happens, the desired food has lost the fabulous once thought that made it special to the individual. Thus, cheat days may be far and few in the long term diet.

Water is Number One!

Water is now the number one drink over soda pop beverages. Why? There has been a decline in drinking soda pop beverages due to the additives that cause adverse reactions, increase amounts of sugar awareness in the various beverages, and the over increasing obesity on the United States.

The decrease in sugar beverages relates to weight loss. Often, individuals find they are not drinking the require amounts of
water per day. The required amount is eight 8 ounces of water per day or 64 ounces total. This equals half a gallon of water. Instead, individuals easily drink a 64 ounce of soda pop beverage with meals.

Providers recommend cutting back or cutting out of sugary drinks. Dieters find that when they cut out these drinks, they lose
weight. Many losing quite a few pounds over several months. Weight loss may be up to twenty pounds as the body's sugar
supply is cut off and the body begins using stores of fat for body requirements instead of instant sugar burns.

Need to lose weight? Consider giving up sugar drinks.

Tip:

Try to drink 8 bottles of water throughout the day. This will help decrease any soda pop beverage but many have trouble doing this. Try drinking one bottle of water then the same amount of soda pop, followed by another bottle of water. Begin adding ice to the soda pop and it will help you wean off the soda pop. The addition of water will help prevent the caffeine headaches. If you feel a headache starting, drink water. Do note that many headache products have caffeine in them. This may cause a rebound caffeine headache, not the soda pop.

Diet Failure

The hard part of diet change is expecting results that may not materialize. Why is this? Is this a true failure of a diet?

The goal of a diet is to lose x pounds in x time. If the weight is not lost in x time, is this a failure? What if weight is
lost but not enough to achieve the goal? The perception of the goal being realistic is half the battle with weight loss.

Example: The goal is to lose one pound a week. This means that the person needs to cut out 250 calories every day to lose
a pound.

This should be an easy goal but the weigh day comes and the pound was not lost. Is this a failure? Yes. To lose the pound but
not why the pound was not lost. There are often other outside circumstances for a pound not being lost.

One reason is women may be menstruating and will gain or hold fluid that will relate in more than one pound gained. Working out and gaining muscle weight will offset any weight in fat lost and may cancel out weight loss on the scale.

Other failures with weight loss can be, while following a low calorie diet, the type of calories eaten may have last longer
in the body creating no change in weight. Types of food in the body do not dissolve in the system as quickly as others, will
remain in the body and keep weight from being realized.

But did you fail? Possibly not but the psychological expectations can make one feel that failure has been obtained and thus
giving up, will cause failure and no weight loss.

When working toward a goal, do not give up on the first try.

Menstruation:

Do not change the workout or diet when menstruating. Note the weight gain but do not fret. Once the menstruation is completed, the weight will drop off along with the weight per diet and exercise. This is not a fail time. This is nature and your body is normal.

Losing Weight and Making It Work

How do you make losing weight work?

1. A clear understanding of how long it is going to take to lose weight normally. Normal weight loss is one to two pounds a week. This is 250 to 500 calories a day omitted from the daily intake.
2. Set a realistic goal. To lose 52 pounds is 52 weeks of losing one pound a week.
3. Do not get discourage. Understand you will still have tomorrow regardless. Things do not happen at internet speeds. Dropping weight too quickly may not stay off or cause other health issues.
4. Retraining the mind and body of what a normal size meal is. At 2,000 calories, a day that is 666.66 calories for three meals. For those who want to blame the Devil regarding dieting, there you go with the numbers. Two meals a day is 1,000 calories and this can add up quickly. While a regular size hamburger is often 500 calories, there is not much room to add on a regular size of 400 to 500 calories of fries. So, two meals like that and you are done for the day.
5. Balance of calories is important. There are three types of calories; carbohydrates, fats, and protein. Typical for 2,000 calories the percentage are 50% carbohydrates, 30% fats, and 20% proteins. Depending on the number of calories, the percentages will adjust accordingly.
6. Realize it will take time to learn about calories and the percentages. It will be a chore and mindfulness at first but will become easier as you progress with your knowledge. It may take several months to get the facts learned that it becomes second nature.
7. Failure happens. Desserts happen. Holidays happen. Two things that can be done. One accept the results for the day and restart the next day. Another option is cut out calories on day two that was over from day one. The trouble with this method is it gets crazy trying to keep the totals correct and may result in malnourishment.
8. Never give up. As long as you are breathing you got a chance at this.

Just a few ways to work on losing weight and moving forward. Be patient and the goal will be achieved.

Losing Weight and the Journey

Often as a provider you have to walk the talk. I can see in the mirror what everyone around me sees. So, what should I do about that? It is hard to tell others how to lose weight and get them to believe you when you are not following your own advice.

Time to follow my own advice. I recommend losing one to two pounds a week. This means that 250 in calories a day omitted from total calories to lose one pound a week and 500 calories for two pounds a week. I recommend under 2,000 calories which is a Federal guideline of calories that need to be consumed per day for a healthy person. Do understand that diabetics may need to be on a lower calorie count per American Diabetic Association recommendations and other specialty needs diets.

First, everyone is on a diet. A diet is your menu of food per day. The total calories for this menu should not go over 2,000 calories. If it is, cutting back to this number may result in losing weight.

Okay, I can do this. I will start eating 2,000 calories a day. I tracked my calories with a cell phone app called myfitnesspal.com. What I liked about this app is it now has a barcoding scanner included to help keep more of an accurate total of calories. It then breaks down those calories into types of calories and nutrients, and the best part it is the standard option is free. Perfect for my research of evidence-based results.

The research project:
The journey started the week after the Christmas holidays.
The entire project would be one year or 52 weeks.
The weight loss goals were at least one pound. Two pounds would be fabulous.
The calorie count was 2,000 per day.

Weigh in would be weekly and nothing but skin. We both already know we carry 5-10 pounds per day of accessories, so to be as accurate as we could, skin was the call on this one.

One of us would just begin cutting back and not tracking calories. The other one would track the food and calories.
A decent research project.

The results of the first quarter or 16 weeks into the project?

After implementing the calorie app, my goal for weight loss of one pound a week was slightly lower than the 2,000 calories. The real shocker came when I begin putting in the calories from my meals. Many takeout meals were way over the totals for the day. Desserts were the totals for the days and added into meals I would normal eat, no wonder I had gained weight.

Downsizing the portions was helpful but still as shocking to find out that many small sizes were full of calories of 500 or more. When you divide the 2,000 by three for three meals, suddenly I was running out of meals per day. I had gone down to one or two meals and was maxing out the calories. Portion sizes where skewed from what I thought was right verses what was right. I started implementing actual measuring tools and trying to figure out just how many calories my hand could hold.

The good thing was I was really eating fairly healthy regarding my choices and percentages per day with carbohydrates, fats and proteins. I did find it easy to cut back on the carbohydrates but increasing the proteins was a struggle. I was just not eating enough protein to help the weight loss. I began looking for higher protein meals to consume. This turned out to be trickery than I thought with take-out menus. Meals I normally considered "man's meals" where suddenly "women's meals" if I wanted to fill hungry and meet my protein goals. After 12 weeks, I began to really notice when I did not have enough protein for the day. I just did not have enough energy. At the end of the day all I could think about was sleeping.

Now my teammate found that cutting back on soda pop and cutting back the sugar in the daily cups of coffee made a huge difference fast. The initial weight loss per week was an easy two pounds by doing this. Once the weight loss had tapered, then portion sizes were scaled back and this kept the two pounds coming off a week.

Then a rough patch of trying to keep the balance in food sources would relate in upset stomachs. Often the only way to resolve with no medications was to just fast for a few meals. The stomach issues would resolve and more careful sections continued. There was just some things that over doing it was beginning not to be worth it. One splurge resulted in several days of agony.

During this time, we began noticing how white food was way too high in sugar and left our joints hurting more than they should. We began cutting out white food. Limiting sandwiches to one slice of bread and increasing the protein. We felt better.

The things that went wrong? Candy. Holiday candy. It was alarming that a bite size piece of candy could have up to 45 to 90 calories in one piece. That two to four pieces equaled 240 calories. Minus the candy calories out of 2,000 left less calories for meals. I began realizing while the candy was wonderful, I would rather have had a hamburger or several slices of bacon instead. It was not much better when I ventured into the new ice cream mixes for the year. I noticed that the serving sizes had gone from ½ to ¾ cups and the calories increased with this. I began comparing two scopes of ice cream to a takeout hamburger. Two scopes were equaling a meal in calories for me. I was not happy. Desserts equal meals. Dessert meals did not quell the hunger and it caused me to go over my calorie count. This resulted in no shows of weight loss for a week.

The last miserable result was something I was born with and that is female hormones. Those weeks were added weight to the scale. The first month was traumatizing to see a few more pounds on the total than losing one pound. I had to keep the faith and stay the course. Hoping that when all was said and done the following week's number would still show a loss. Happily, to report that the female hormone weight did come off and the one pound I was fighting to come off with it. The spikes in my weight loss showed a regular adventure in being a female. A few months into the one pound a week and I was not as traumatized when I saw a spike. I did have to be extra mindful to not let hormones do the talking when it came time to eating.

After 16 weeks, good results. We have lost weight. Total weight loss so far has been 38 pounds. Now this is fabulous but I have to not beat myself up on my share of the contribution. I am off a few pounds of the goal. I have to say it was the one too many days over my calorie count goals that resulted in no shows on the scales. My partner has also noticed the 2 pounds slipping to 1.5 pounds on average now and he's really cut back on portion sizes to keep the weight loss going.

While to each other we do not look a whole lot different and others have not really noticed, we are seeing some progress in trying to keep our pants up now. Clothes are getting a little baggy and double chins and muffin tops are starting to thin out a bit.

Other things we have noticed is we have to get sleep. We need so many hours a day of sleep to function and need to keep the protein up to keep the mind functioning at high capacity. Lowering the carbohydrates has made the need for arthritis pain medication limiting as well. Very important since we live in Ohio where the weather changes every five minutes and you feel it in your joints and bones.

It has also been hard to stay positive with only losing one to two pounds a week. It is so frustrating to look in the mirror and not see the amazing difference. This is why taking a picture weekly would be a good idea. Easier to look back at photos to see the differences. We have not been taking pictures but looking back over the YouTube and business pictures, we can see some differences that hare happening.

Looking forward:
After four months of trying to stay under 2,000 calories, we have learned a lot. Marketing and advertisement has derailed what we think is the right portions size. We now pay attention more to the calories on menu boards. We notice that small sizes are not options in some

areas. Condiments can be an extra 100-200 calories not included in a meal. We found one chicken sandwich with an added 200 calories just because it had mayo on it. We also have discovered the excessive hidden amounts of sugar in food. Things we normally would not think had sugar in them. There has been a lot of unlearning and relearning what a portion size is. What is really considered healthy and what is not.

We will keep going with our research. This December we will complete our one pound a week goal. Some days it seems like a long way off and other days, it seems like it will be here quickly. If we keep up the one pound a week goal, we will both lose 52 pounds for a total of 104 pounds. So far, we are down 38 of those total pounds. Very exciting team effort thus far.

The 52 weeks goal is almost complete as volume #4 is going to the publishers.

2018 "Team Goins" will release their diets and how well they did.

- What worked and what did not.
- How much did they lose?
- How much exercise did they do?
- Did they have any setbacks?
- Did they get sick during the year and did that hurt the diet?
- What did the weekly weight equal to?
- What did they eat?
- What apps did they use?
- How many sizes did they lose?
- Did they cook or eat out?
- Did they cheat?
- Did they take any pictures?

Losing Weight and Frustration of Speed

The first part of losing weight is being realistic. Marketing and advertisement over the years has taught us non-realistic ideas of how fast we can lose weight and what we should look like when we do lose weight.

The realistic losing weight of 1-2 pounds a week is normal and to be expected. Monthly weight loss is 4-8 pounds. This means that a person is very over weight, will need to understand that the weight loss is going to take more than a couple weeks, months, but maybe several years.

One pound a week x 52 weeks is 52 pounds a year.
Two pounds a week x 52 weeks is 104 pounds a year.
104 x 2 years is 208 pounds.
104 x 3 years is 312 pounds.
104 x 4 years is 416 pounds.
104 x 5 years is 520 pounds.

Setting realistic goals and understanding this is going to take some time, helps keep a person from getting frustrated from the speed of how long it takes to lose weight. Remember, this typically didn't happen yesterday that the body is overweight.

The body is not going to magically lose all the weight tomorrow.
Understanding that a major weight loss is going to take 12 months or longer and it is ongoing. There will be many temptations along the way that will have to be adverted to stay on track or decisions on how to limit the temptations or change those items out for lower calories to stay on track will be the choice.

A good mindset and established goals can help an individual to be successful. Remember, do or not, the individual has a choice and it is their responsibility. The hand can go to the mouth or not. Each day is a challenge but those days will add up and the person's choices will be reflected in their body.

Losing Weight and Nutrition Labels

The nutrition labels are based off a percentage of the daily recommended 2,000 calories. This means that every food label has a percentage that is broken down into what the food is and how much of the food needs to be eaten to get the equation of a serving size.

Right here, this thought that can toss many over the edge because they do not understand what a serving size or the information presented means. The label on the side of nearly every packaged item of food has a white label and information. The label will begin with what it is and what a serving size is. Each container of food may have more than one serving size in it. The serving size is an amount of food that is counted or weighed out. The container may have a total weight and list more than one serving size.

The amount of what a serving size can be quite shocking to an individual. They may not realize the amount they have been eating is one serving. It may be more or less. This adjustment can be corrected and help an individual add or gain weight.
The serving size is equal to an amount of food of x number of calories. This serving is then subtracted from the daily recommended amount of 2,000 calories.

Example: 24 green onion potato chips equals 150 calories. Subtracted 150 calories from 2,000 total calories for the day and the individual has 1,850 more calories for the day to eat.
Every calorie is divided into three components of carbohydrates, proteins, and fats.

The information on the label will break down into percentages of how many carbohydrates, proteins, and fats are listed per serving size. Why is this important? Because even if some individual eats all the same type of food, such as 2,000 carbohydrates, the body will react to it. The body like a car. Putting the wrong gas in, not having enough gas, or a flat tire, and the car will not go. The body is the same. The body needs a percentage of each type of calories to make the body function properly. By eating the correct amounts the body will then not be sluggish, have energy, and handle the daily tasks better.

Once an individual can manage a 2,000-calorie diet per day, the next challenge is to look at the types of calories ingested and eat accordingly to the percentages. Many will find that limiting their carbohydrates and increasing their protein will help build muscle and result in fat weight loss. Fatigue will diminish and the body will have more energy.

Losing Weight 2,000 Calories Diet

A diet is what we call your menu for eating daily. It has taken on a new meaning with media and marketing to mean that when you are "on a diet" you are losing weight.

A 2,000-calorie diet is a total of 2,000 calories per day.

Reasons for dieting:
Occasions coming up in the future and you wish to look fabulous.
Finding out that your health has changed and it is needed to loss or gain weight.
A person just cannot do the things they use to do because of their weight.

Whatever the decision to lose weight, you have to start somewhere, and most folks announce they are on a diet now.
What is a "diet"? A diet then becomes a certain food to eat or not, an amount of food consumed, and other food changes.

Types of changes:

1. Decrease in carbohydrates. Food with high carbohydrates are white foods of bread, pasta, and pastries.
2. Increase in fruits and vegetables. This may go from not eating any fruit or vegetable, to eating this type of food during the day to keep up blood sugar and energy levels.
3. Proteins may need to increase. This may be hard if the individual has omitted this or cannot afford this. Eggs, Chicken, fish, pork, and beef may need to be increased in the diet. Other options are peanut butter, beans, and nuts.
4. Omit snack foods and sweets from the diet. Often, this is where many find hidden calories or where their diet has gone askew. Many times, just omitting these foods will reflect in weight loss.

The calories from each type of food are totaled up per day to equal 2,000. This is when the shocker of just how many calories many individuals are eating per day is a problem. Reflection in over the top of the daily recommendation for everyone of 2,000 calories may be found in one take out meal and then some. Many establishments have calories listed on their menu boards or websites. It can be quite alarming to find out how many calories has been ingested in a single meal when trying to stay under 2,000 calories.

While the recommendations is 2,000 calories per day, an individual may already be eating healthy and targeted in on this number for a long time. They may not be seeing any results in the change of their weight. Then, lower the total of calories may help. Diabetic diets are 1,200 to 1,600 calories and this change in total calories may be just enough to help shed 1-2 pounds a week. To lose 1-2 pounds a week, the daily omit of 250-500 calories must be done.

It can be quite interesting to go from having no idea to watching what 2,000 calories in a diet is per day. When trying to begin dieting, begin focusing on omitting food to reach 2,000 calories.

This is followed by re-arranging the type of calories ingested. Individuals will begin noticing that omitting the sweets, sugars, and high carbohydrates will help them feel better. Some may struggle to change the food sources ingested due to the pickiness of their eating and may need to learn to like new food sources to replace the other types ingested.

Eating 2,000 calories daily will be a challenge to some but remember that every day restarts and so will your chance to begin again.

Alternative calorie diets:

It is not recommended that one should go under 1,000 calories as it causes the body to go into starvation.

- 1,000 (Two meals of 500 calories)
- 1,200 (Two meals of 600 calories)
- 1,500 (Three meals of 500 calories)
- 1,800 (Three meals of 600 calories)
- 2,000 (Three meals of 667 calories)

Meat:

Roast beef 4 oz is 192 calories

Tuna 4 oz is 209 calories

Hamburger 4 oz raw, ground, 70% lean is 376 calories

Steak 4 oz is 307 calories

5 Ways to Walk 5,000

Easy to say do standard 10,000 steps a day. It is actually harder to do them daily. Especially if you have been living a very sedentary lifestyle. Like every elephant you have to eat, it begins with one bite.

1. Figure out how many steps are 5,000. The average human's steady walk equals 2,000 steps a mile and 5,000 steps equals approximately 2.5 miles.
2. Miles is not a lot of walking when you figure in all the walking you do from the time you get out of bed to the time you go back to bed. A good day of cleaning the house will equate to a mile of steps inside.
3. Fitting in walking when we as society have become very efficient at multitasking. Ways to increase walking; walk to work and back, walk to talk to someone instead of messaging them, and walk around the block, or go to a local mall and walk.
4. Download a free pedometer for your cell phone. It can keep track of your steps and may include a calorie counter.
5. Involve a buddy to walk with you or walk a path where you can say "hi" to people or enjoy nature. Daily walks will have you noticing the world and the people around you more.

The average city block is about 16 to 17 blocks per mile or approximately 250 acers.

A football field is 300 feet by 160 feet or 1.1. acres.

Sedentary: under 5,000 steps per day

Low activity: 5,001 to 7,499 steps per day

Activity: 7,500 to 10,000 steps

Very Activity: 10,000 steps +

Exercise in What You Have

As a society, we are drilled into having the right gear or tool for the right thing and this is awesome if you have the space and money to make this happen. Not everyone has the space or the money to go shopping for exercising clothing. Some of us are not even the right size to buy the exercising clothing to wear. What do we do? We exercise in what we have.

1. Shoes are big deal with any exercise. A pair of sneakers with support will do fine until they wear out. Odds are, there is a pair of sneakers in your closet or under your bed right now that will do just fine.
2. A tee shirt or regular shirt of any color or design will be fine. If you are exercising at night, it will need to be light in color or reflective to oncoming lights.
3. Shorts or light pants to wear will help keep the thighs from rubbing together and meet the needs in varies weather. Pockets can carry cells, keys, and ID.
4. Under garments. Support and not binding is the key here. Keeping everything in place without it jiggling around is helpful when exercising.
5. Less focus on the what to wear will help you focus on the exercise. It will help you find less excusing on exercising.

> Why wear what you have?
>
> Sometimes going and buying clothes to work out can motivate or devastate you.
>
> If you are on a budget, then wearing what you have is a good choice. The clothes will begin to get big and you will be replacing them with smaller clothes.
>
> Safety with wearing clothes you already have is a good idea. Sometimes not bringing attention to your activities in an area that is not safe is a good idea. Always keep alert in your surroundings.
>
> Do be sure you wear clothes that others can see. Wearing black in early morning darkness makes it hard to see you.
>
> Always carry a cell phone if possible if you should need to call for help.

Do You Know Your Sugar Calories?

One of the most wonderful things that is discovered when using a calorie counter is, just what is in the food we are eating. One of the biggest surprises is how much sugar are in the items we are consuming.

Sugar is in high volumes in many of the foods we are eating and a calorie counter can rat them out in food really quickly.

The Arthritis Foundation states excessive sugar in the diet can cause inflammation in the body. It can cause the joints to hurt and add on pounds. Limiting the sugar can limit the inflammation in the body.

Sugar breaks down into natural sugars and added sugars. Natural sugars are in fruits and milk and added sugars are products added to anything to make it sweet.

So how much sugar should we eat per day?

The American Heart Association recommends;

Men should eat less than 9 teaspoons of sugar or 36 grams equaling 150 calories per day.

Women should eat less than 6 teaspoons of sugar or 25 grams equaling 100 calories a day.

2017 Sugar Prices:

US Raw Sugar: 27.83 cents per pound

US Refined Sugar: 30.7 cents per pound

US Retail Sugar: 64.7 center per pound

One pound of raw sugar is 87.09 teaspoons of sugar

9 teaspoons of sugar x 31 days = 279 teaspoons of sugar divided by 87.09 = 3.2 bags of sugar per month eaten by men. (150 x 9 x 31 =41,850 calories)

6 teaspoons of sugar x 31 days = 186 teaspoons of sugar divided by 87.09 = 2.1 bags of sugar eaten per month by women. (100 x 6 x 31 = 18,600)

A husband and wife would eat 5.3 bags of sugar a month or 63.6 bags of sugar a year. (41,850 + 18,600= 60,450 calories month/520,800 calories a year)

Three Cheap Calories for a Full Belly

Financially it is hard to watch calories and diet at the same time. Some things are expensive. How can you keep your belly full and watch the calories?

1. Eggs are a wonderful source of protein and low in calories. There is a hundred ways to make them that eggs will never get dull. The easiest way to make eggs is to buy a dozen of eggs. Boil all of them, remove the shells, and put them in containers for on the go meals. One egg is approximately 90 calories. Two or three in a baggie is a protein meal on the go. One dozen of eggs can make up to 4 meals.
2. Peanut butter is another option for a quick on the go meal. One tablespoon of peanut butter is approximately 200 calories. A peanut butter spoon works well for the hungry and busy person on the go.
3. Water is the prefect replacement for any beverage. No sugars or modified chemicals and replacing two beverages with water daily can save up to 500 calories a day resulting in one to two pounds lost a week.

Note:

Do note that one saltine cracker has 45 calories. A packet of 2 saltine crackers is 90 calories.

A sleeve of crackers holds approximately 40 crackers.

One tablespoon of peanut butter with two crackers is 290 calories.

Fasting to Lose Weight

Many will find that if they stop eating after a particular time of the day that this will result in weight loss for them. This is called fasting. Fasting is when you stop eating for the day and breaking fast or breakfast is the first meal of the next day. Marketing has done a good job of associating breakfast as the first meal of the day. Breaking fast can really be at any time of the day since it is the first meal that is eaten for the day. If the first meal of the day is in the afternoon, then that is the breaking fast meal. To many this is not breakfast but lunch or a noon day meal.

Will fasting help you lose weight? Yes, it can help you lose weight. It can help your body focus on the current food and resources within the body. It can help prevent food behaviors that result in gaining weight.

The last meal of the day begins the fast until the next day. Adding hours between meals can help with weight loss. Many find that eating the last meal by six o'clock and not eating to the next day at six o'clock will give 12 hours of fasting. This is enough time for the body to process the food eaten and prevent weigh gain. Excessive or long-term fasting can result in the body breaking down and cause wasting resulting in illness or death.

Breaking Fast is the first meal of the day.

Breaking fast can be done at any time. If the first meal of the day is at noon, then this is breaking fast meal.

Breakfast is the shorten version of breaking fast and was advertised as the first meal of the day in the 1970's. It is currently accepted that breakfast is a morning meal and is eaten of particular foods; such as eggs, pancakes, waffles, biscuits and gravy, sausage, and cold/hot cereals served with toast, orange juice, and milk.

Breakfast foods may be eaten at other times of the day but may not be offered due to cooking times of other products or request for different foods.

Eating Too Much?

The average diet recommended is 2,000 calories a day. It can be very surprising to go out to eat and realize your entire meal in one sitting is over the 2,000 calories a day recommended. This is a good place to start in realizing how to cut back to 2,000 calories. Many consuming over 2,000 calories will see the scales shift in weight loss by just cutting to 2,000 calories.

The next step is taking 2,000 calories and breaking it into more than one meal per day. Society eats a morning meal, a noon meal, and an evening meal. This meals that the 2,000 calories should be divided by 3 meals and the calories per meal should be 667 calories or divided by 2 meals and this is 1,000 calories.

Adjusting to two or three meals spread out through the day instead of one meal of 2,000 calories can help the body feel less hungry. This major adjustment of cutting back will result in weight loss.

<table>
<tr><td>

Typically at least one meal a day is the meal with the most calories. This may be a noon meal for those working early morning jobs, such as farming, cattle, or chickens. Others may eat their heaviest meal in the evening hours after the day is completed. This may result in difficulty with weight loss or GI upset as the night progresses.

</td></tr>
</table>

Cutting Back from 2,000 Calories to Lose Weight.

The recommended calories per day is 2,000. Many will find they are eating over that amount and need to cut back to 2,000. Once they do, they find they are losing weight. Then they adjust to spreading the calories out into two or three meals per day and find the hunger is not as bad.

Once reaching the 2,000 calories and not seeing any weight loss on the scale, it is time to cut back calories. The Diabetic Association recommends two diets of 1,600 and 1,200 to help manage diabetes.

A 2,000-calorie diet in two meals is 1,000 calories or 667 for three meals a day.
A 1,600-calorie diet in two meals is 800 calories or 533 for three meals a day. (2000-1600=400 calories)
A 1,200-calorie diet in two meals is 600 calories or 400 calories for three meals a day. (2000-1400=600 calories)

The loss of 250 calories a day will result in one pound of weight loss per week.

The loss of 500 calories a day will result in two pounds of weight loss per week.

www.AmericanDiabeticAssoiation.org

1,200 calories

1,600 calories

Diabetics may need to test their blood sugars before and after meals to see if additional medications are needed.

Your provider can check a hemoglobin Alc. This is 120 days of your blood cells collecting sugar. If the Alc is over 6.5 -7.0 depending on your age, you may need medication. If your Alc is over 9.0 you may need insulin added to your medications.

Drink God's Soda Pop?

Water is God's Soda Pop. Currently, there is no patent on water. God still retains this patent. It is the number one soda pop in the world. It is also very good for you. Yet, how much water should you drink? One good way to figure this out is to see how much "water" you are putting out of your body. The biggest gauge of water is called urine. The color of the urine is diluted by water.

If the urine is very dark in color, then there is not enough water in the body to dilute the urine. Increasing the water intake, will dilute the urine and the urine will lighten up in color. The goal for urine color is light yellow. This means the urine has been diluted with enough water.

How much "water" does the body hold? The bladder typically holds 400 mls before the urge to the bathroom is present. This approximately one 16-ounce bottle of water. The bladder makes 30 to 60 mls an hour of urine. Roughly one to two shot glasses of urine.

The recommended drinking rule of thumb is eight 8 ounces of water per day. Now here is the catch. Per day. Per day means 24 hours. A lot of people will say they can't drink that much water. Dividing the 24-hour day up, this will mean that you need to drink 8 ounces of water every 3 hours. Of course, there is supposed to be sleep of 8 hours per day, so minus the 8 from 24 hours and that is 16 hours per day. Thus, 16 hours divided by 8 would be drinking water every 2 hours per day.

Not to terrible to have to drink that much water but this is a rule of thumb not required. Sometimes this may be too much water as the urine is already diluted or not enough in the summer due to sweating the water out and not urinating it.

No matter how you divide It up, God's soda pop is good for you.

Bragging Rights!

The City of Hamilton, Ohio has the best tap water in the world! This means that water right out of the faucet is the best here!

Plateau a Diet

Ugh! I have not lost any weight or the scales has not budged. This is called plateauing. It can last a lot longer than we want because it means we have reached the equal amount of intake to outtake in our diets and exercise.

This means we have to do something to shake it up, change what we are doing, or add something.

The easiest is to add more exercising, change the workout style, or increase the time and effort exercising. Perhaps taking the stairs instead of the elevator? Parking farther way from the door? Walking to tell someone something instead of messaging them?

The hardest is reviewing the diet to see what can be eliminated or changed up. Reviewing the calorie intake, can it be changed or lowered? Can protein increase or decrease? Sugars removed? Daily sugar intake should only be 150 calories for men and 100 calories for women.

The next problem is realizing that plateauing may happen long before one realizes it has happened. It may be several weeks of working hard on exercising and eating with no results showing up on the scales. This can be frustrating and can change motivation.

Yet, the next time you plateau, realize it is really reaching your goal you set. This means that the goal needs to be adjusted to reach the real end goal wished. The set goals may need to be reset many times to reach the wish goal desired.

> Plateau is when your weight goal has not changed for 3-4 weeks. If you have not changed your weight in two weeks you may be starting to plateau. This is a good time to implement another exercise, change it up, or restrict your diet.

No Diet Support

Eventually one has to realize that they are all in or not. It is not about anyone but you. There may not be support or help with your diet. Should there be? It comes down to it is your responsibility and your fault on the outcomes, good or bad. The motion of hand to mouth is your reasonability. No one else has this responsibility for you.

No support may not be a bad thing because weight loss takes time and a lot longer than most dieters want to admit. Losing 100 pounds is a big goal. Breaking it down into 25 pound goals is 4 major dieting goals. Reaching one, then the next is easier to realize than working on the straight 100 pounds to lose.

Example:
250 pounds. Goal for BMI is 150 pounds. This means there is 25 pound goals of 225, 200, 175, and then 150 pounds.

The other realization is it takes a long time to lose weight. On average if you cut out 250 calories per day out of the diet or exercised to burn 250 calories, this is only one pound a week. There are 52 weeks in a year and this means it will take 52 weeks to lose 52 pounds. If you increase the loss of calories to 500 per day for 52 weeks then this is 104 pounds.

The real problem here is that it may take a year to lose the weight or longer. The mindset for the long term needs to be realized before success can be effective and sometimes depending on long term support may not be a realistic idea. Support has to come from within to maintain the goal.

Setting the mind to understand the goal is long term will help one to feel the self-support needed.

Diet Logs:

A diet log is a good support of how well you are doing. Periodically look back at your success and cheer yourself on.

Cheering yourself on is good for your self-esteem. Give yourself pep talks. "You can do this." "You are awesome." "We didn't think we could do it but we did." "(Your name) I am proud of you!"

Stay in Bed and Exercise

Too lazy to move? Don't want to get out of bed? Weather is too bad to exercise? Stay in bed! What? Yes! Stay in bed! You can exercise while in bed!

Exercises to do while in bed:
Crunches
Flutter kicks
Planking
Push-ups

The bed offers advantages to those who are not able to get down on the floor and do exercises. It will also help sway fears of not being able to get up or smashing your face into the floor while doing pushups or planking.

The disadvantage is the bed may be a bit soft and more strength may be needed to do some of the exercises but that is all good too.

Bed exercises work great for a lot of folks who are too frail to get up and move, those who do not have time to go to a gym and work out, or folks with days so jam packed that only some crunches in bed is all they have time to do.

Sit ups

Do not underestimate the sit up in bed. Sure it is hard to reach those knees but eventually you will reach them. It may take months for it to happen but if you do them every day, it will be a habit you just do. You will even feel weird if you skip them after a while. So hop back into bed and do them. Those "abds" will show up. They might be hidden under some fat rolls but they are there waiting for their big day to show off. One day you will look in the mirror and they will be looking back. Do not give in and do not give up. This is just what you do now.

Exercise on Breaks at Work

An 8-hour work day involves 30 minutes for lunch and two breaks. Why not take one or both breaks to get some exercise in? Maybe even get a co-worker or all of them to join you?

Ideas to implement:

Planking for a minute
Pushups
Up and down a flight of stairs
Walk around the office outside
Arm circles
Spelling out the alphabet with your arms and legs

Did you know that if you exercise 15 minutes every day for 4 days you will have exercised for one hour? If you exercise on both 15-minute breaks for 4 days, you will have exercised two hours. Toss in the fifth day with exercise on both breaks and exercising time gained is two and half hours!

It is a lot easier to exercise than you think!

Hate meetings as much as I do?

Do standing meetings. Everyone has to stand for the meeting and hit the main points.

Really hate meetings. Do plank meetings. Either everyone planks or there is no need for a meeting.

The corporate world gets hung up on meetings and can kill a lot of time this way.

If you are in a meeting, stand up every 15 minutes and stretch. Give your tush a rest.

Working in Exercise in Your Day?

Did you know that you are exercising all the time? Exercise is movement of the body. Just getting up and walking around your own home, you will get a few steps in per day.

Another way to measure the steps in a day is with a pedometer. A pedometer can be attached to your shoe or you can download an application that you can put on your cell phone.

100 steps walked is half a city block. At Couture Health Care, one patient will walk at least half of one city block during the course of their visit and not realize they have. Just an example how easy it is to walk without realizing you are going very far.

Based on the average steps of per person, 200 steps will be one block. Twenty blocks or 2,000 steps equal one mile. On average, if you walk 20 city blocks you have walked one mile.

It will be interesting to find your baseline to see how many steps you really are walking per day. Aren't you curious now? You may be walking miles and not realize it.

<table><tr><td>

Walking:

Most folks have no idea how far they walk per day. Download any free app to count steps on your cell phone or get a tracker for your shoe/hip to wear.

Your goal is 5,000 steps per day to be active.

</td></tr></table>

Time to Exercise?

The first part of exercising is taking the time to do it. This can be very difficult when you realize that you already need an extra 24 hours in your day. Now you have to fit in an exercise program?

Right here is where many folks will toss in the towel on even starting exercising. Don't get discouraged. There are ways to exercise in your day that don't require going to a gym every day for 1-2 hours.

1. Walk to work. Is your place of work a mile away? Now is the time to start walking there.
2. An hour lunch? Go for 30 minutes instead of lounging like androconia after you eat.
3. Office up on the fifth floor? Take the stairs instead of the elevators.
4. Afternoon break is afternoon snack time? Go for a walk instead of eating a snack to refresh.
5. Work from home? Go walk around the block several times to clear you head and get some sunshine.

Some ideas to get you started and many will realize that they can add exercise into their daily life without much fuss of having to get a gym membership.

Inside Walking:

There are times when you just can't get outside to walk. Walk inside. Walk to your bedroom to your kitchen and back. Walk around the coffee table or kitchen table.

Walk during commercials on the television.

Walk during songs on the radio.

Walk for 30 minutes inside and keep walking until the time is up.

Exercising and Neighborhood Watch

There are a lot of good reasons that you should get out and walk in your neighborhood. One reason is getting necessary exercise in the day. The other reason is to have a neighborhood watch system. Neighborhood watch systems are when the neighbors watch out for each other and their things. Keeping "shoppers" from removing things from the neighborhood, causing a bad rap on the corners with soliciting products and services, and bringing housing prices down.

Freelancing entrepreneurs, who work the neighborhood or the corners, may be easily persuaded to relocate to a new location when the neighborhood is active in their area. Too many folks walking, running, biking, mowing, and playing in their yards, sends notice that the location isn't a profitable one or a safe one to freelance work.

In addition to keeping the neighborhood safe, the individuals will get to see and recognize the people in their neighborhood. It will help build up housing market prices and keep turnover of selling homes down in the neighborhood because the neighbors will want to stay where it is safe and feels like home.

<table>
<tr><td>

Neighborhood Watch:

By walking at the same time outside, your area becomes known for too many folks out and about.

If you see something that isn't the norm for your area, call your local authorities. Your calls are recorded and trouble areas are brought to attention to the local governments.

When walking, do wear visible clothing and keep your cell ready to use.

Wave at everyone you pass. This draws attention to you and your area. Criminals don't like friendly people and nosey neighbors.

</td></tr>
</table>

Too Tired to Exercise When I Get Home Exercises

Getting home is the most rewarding part of the day for many folks but many of us need to get in a bit more movement before we settle for the day.

1. Do not sit down when you first come home. Walk around your entire house and in each room first. This will add steps to your day. It will also make sure your home is safe and there were no problems while away.
2. Grab the leash and take the pets for a walk. You know it was forever since they saw you last.
3. Walk around the house with the cat food before putting it down. It will improve your coordination trying not to be tripped and get your cat use to the routine before they are fed.
4. Leave the homework for later. Get outside with the kids for you and them time for 15 minutes. Walk, run, jump, and more outside then come in and start the evening at home.
5. Greet your love one! Stand, hold them, hug them, and talk with them. Touch is a wonderful form of releasing hormones that improve mood and gives you valuable time together.
6. Go to bed. Give yourself a bedtime and stick to it. Okay, maybe not the same bedtime you had when you were a kid but an adult bedtime. This will give you more energy and help relieve tiredness.

Options:

Take a nap when you get home and then set your alarm to get up later to go to gym.

Do a quick set of push-ups, sit-ups, or short walk when you get home.

Plank for a minute before eating and after.

Do sitting exercises. Circles with your arms, flutter kicks with your feet, and ABCs spelled out as you sit.

I Sit at My Desk All Day Exercises.

Some jobs require attachment to a desk, telephone, or keyboard to earn a living. Exercise can still be done while sitting.

1. First pick a time. Top of the hour, every 15 minutes, or after every telephone call is answered.
2. Take a can of food or beverage and hold it over your head with both hands. Then slowly let your hands and can fall behind your head. Repeat until the time is up or another call comes in.
3. Every time you are on hold while on the telephone, stick your legs out straight in front of you and raise them up and down. This is called a flutter kick in swimming. Do it until someone starts taking.
4. Every time someone comes in your office, stand up. Not only is it professional but it keeps the bum from falling asleep.
5. Arms out straight and do arm circles after the boss leaves your area for three minutes.
6. One hour before quitting time, take slow deep breaths in and out for two minutes. Do arm circles and leg circles for two minutes each limb. This will help wake up the body for going home and give a little zest at the end of the day.
7. At break times, do ten squats to help keep the circulation going.
8. Wear a pedometer at work to see how many steps you are getting in per day and then try to get up and walk around a little to add to it. You will be surprised at how many steps you may be really getting in.

<table>
<tr><td>

Change it up

Sit on an exercise ball.

Stand at your desk.

Stand up every 15 minutes and stretch.

Go outside or stand by the window to get fresh air.

Do flexing of the fingers, hands, arms, and legs.

</td></tr>
</table>

I'm Not Old Back, Knee, and Feet Exercises.

Life happens and when it does, it can leave us with pain in our backs, knees, and feet. This may lead us to not be able to do the things we use to do, like exercises. What can we do then?

1. When walking with assistance of any cane, walker, or other magical wizard staff; put your foot on the ground heel first. If there is any neuropathy of the foot, it will start in the toes and work back to the heel. This means when you put your foot on the ground toes first you may not feel the ground. This may cause a fall. By putting the heel first on the ground, this aligns the heel with the knee, and then the hip. This supports the lower back and keeps the body upright. Remember not to set off any magical discharges of the staff as it is set down with each step.
2. When standing with assistance, move as far as you can and take a rest. Each day, try for a few more steps. When you think you are done, do one more in honor of your loved one. By the end of each year, you will have done 365 one more steps for them.
3. Sitting exercises will include holding the arms out and doing arm circles to music. Add some friends and books on tape to listen to instead of music may keep the exercises going longer. Certainly, changes the idea of the typical book club weekly meetings. Can you imagine the excitement of horror to the latest flaming sex book? Might even want to wear a saturation finger monitor to see whose heart is racing the most!
4. Want to learn a new language? While sitting move the legs out in the shape of numbers and count. The exercise will help reinforce learning the language and improve coordination.
5. Get up and get down. A newer version of musical chairs. Get up out of your chair and sit down in another chair. Reach around it and pick up or move stuff. Then get up and move to another sitting area. End of game when you make it to the bathroom and sit on the commode.

Morbid Overweight Exercises

The standard is what is called Body Mass Index. It is basically how tall verses how much you weigh equals a percentage. This percentage then falls into too skinny, just right, overweight, obese, and morbid obese.

What happens when you fall in the morbid obese classification? This is typically a person who has trouble dressing, putting on shoes, difficultly with sexual activities, and moving about. Walking is difficult and they will need to sit to rest. Stairs is near impossible. Eventually just moving becomes a problem.

How would one do exercises? First moving is going to be exercise. Simple things, like getting dress will be exercises for many. Thus, time to start is today.

1. Stop letting anyone around you get it for you. You will walk to the kitchen, get up and find things, and move every hour.
2. Begin doing arm circles with hands out, thumbs up or down during all commercials seen or heard. Commercial time is typically two minutes and two seconds. Upon watching television one hour, you will do 15 minutes of arm circles. Four hours will result in one hour of arm circle exercise.
3. Raise legs and do A, B, C with each leg during songs or commercials. Songs on average are three to four minutes. Hardcore leg raises to the song *Frankenstein* is approximately eleven minutes.
4. Stairs. Start trying to get your feet on them and move up them. See how many you can go up and then back down. If you did one or two, excellent. Keep going until you reach the top of the stairs and complete one entire flight. Do this each day.
5. Remember from the *Karate Kid*'s training wax on and wax off? You are going to go into the bathroom and take a washcloth with soap and water and do circle motions on your body. Cover as much as your body as you can then repeat with a wet cloth. Then, repeat a third time with a dry towel. Besides the obvious of cleaning yourself, you will stimulate cell and circulation of your immune system. This will help prevent skin from breaking down, firming up, and improve your overall dexterity. It will also help you keep aware of your body and should any sores be present, check with your provider for treatment options.
6. Reward yourself by standing in front of the mirror and smiling. You did it! Each day, repeat and keep adding as much as you can do.

Your Food Diary Speaks Volumes

Now that you have your daily log/diary app working, focused on your serving sizes, it is now time to look at the calories per day. How many calories are you eating per day? Yes, Uncle Sam recommends 2,000 calories a day but he is averaging every American into a lump sum and estimating that 2,000 calories for everyone should be good. Then, he is dividing serving sizes by the calories per product. This is when you will realize that the tub of ice cream is all the calories for the day. Not an appetizer.

Yet, men, woman, and children all need different levels of calories per day to function. The adjustment in those calories come when the individual is trying to gain, lose, or maintain weight. The number of calories will have to change to accommodate.

There are different numbers of calories per type of diet. Each diet may focus on a particular type of food or lack of food to get a desired effect. Some diets may need to be low in sugar, carbohydrates, or sodium/salt. Other diets may need to be high in potassium, magnesium, and protein. Each individual will find that standard 2,000 calorie diets may not reflect their needs.

The next goal will be to discern what you wish to accomplish. If you wish to lose weight, then you will need to review the diary of food logs to see how many calories in what types of food that is in excess and begin restricting those foods to lower servings or calorie counts.

Sometimes it will be obvious of what the problem food will be. Many will find that drinking regular soda pop has 100-200 calories per serving. Just restricting this intake may result in weight loss to the goal wish to achieve. Others may find that this isn't their problem. They may find that bread every meal is where calories are sneaking in. Cutting out bread every meal may be the cure to losing weight.

Those that need to gain weight may find adding a supplement with minerals, vitamins, and high protein is the solution to putting on the pounds and giving them energy.
What does your food diary say about you?

What to Do with Your Food Diary and Serving Sizes.

Once you have logged or written down your food you have eaten for several days, you will begin to see a pattern. You may see you love bread. Lots of it. Like you would take a semi driver of a bread company hostage if you had to give it up bread person. You may realize you drink way more beverages that you thought. Cases of soda pop, beer, and boxes/bottles of wine and you question if you are recycling the product waste enough. Should you really have two recycling bins larger than your regular garbage bin? You might even realize you really are eating healthy but way too much healthy. Perhaps eating the entire case of strawberries in one sitting isn't a good thing?

Excess in any area is your weakness. Now you have a good idea, if you didn't before, of what food or drink is your kryptonite.

Next look at the number of calories for each meal and each day. This may take a bit of looking up on the internet for nutritional facts about your food. Are you eating a serving size? Do you even know what a serving size is? Yes, the entire tub of ice cream is a serving size but the nutritional information may beg to differ on what a serving size is and it wasn't the entire tub of ice cream.

Serving sizes are huge blows to diets. Huge blows in realizing that you ate ALL the serving sizes and not the recommended sizes. Get out the measuring cups, spoons, and scale to weigh and measure your food first. No, measuring sizes? Any dollar store will have cheap ones you can pick up. Next begin measuring out your food. Take pictures of your sizes. Instagram them if you wish. What will happen is over time you will begin training your eyes that your stomach has been lying to you for years. Your stomach can be perfectly happy with the recommended serving sizes.

Make measuring your food a daily effort and you will begin to realize you didn't need to hold the semi driver hostage for the entire truck of bread. A couple loaves and you can survive.

Food Diaries and Food Logs.

A large majority of people have no idea how to diet or what that means. Many folks won't think they are eating wrong or bad. Many folks may still be eating like they were taught when they were children and not merged to an adult diet.

How do you even know where to start if you do not have any education on diets? What should you do?

The first thing you want to do is begin logging your food intake. All of your food intake. Now it will be a bit overwhelming to have to write down everything you put in your mouth but this is where you will find out what is causing too much weight or too little weight gain or loss.

A diary of food will be ongoing from here until you get a real comfortable idea of looking at food and seeing the calorie content instead of the mindless yummy, eyes rolling back in your head like a shark food fest.

Writing everything down will show you how many portions, calories, and if you are eating a good mix of food or not. Maybe you really are eating healthy but healthy enough for a miniature circus car with twenty midgets healthy amount.
There are lots of way to log your diary. Paper and pencil, calendar apps, or food logger apps.

You can't go wrong in your way of doing it, you just have to start. This is the first step in figuring out what your weakness and your nutrition problem is.

Captain's log...

Document on computers, laptops, tablets, cells, and even paper.

Remember to do it after you eat as later in the day you might just forget that piece of candy or bite of cookie...nope, you ate the entire cookie...and note it in your log.

This is your starship as you are made out of star dust, make sure your hull (body) remains intact and healthy. If not your di-lithium crystals (engine) won't have enough energy to get things done.

Fat Girl Pants Don't Fit Anymore!

There will come a point during the weight loss time when you just can't keep wearing the same baggy clothes any more. It can be very frightening to go shopping. Especially when you already know you are wearing size 22 and 3XL for years. You know right where to go in the store, which rack to look through, and what your options are. You even know what your price for clothing will be. This is the norm. It is comfortable and while you weren't happy about the size and selection, you knew this was the section where you got your clothing.

Now that you are meeting your weight loss goals, the world is scary again. You have no idea what size you are, where you go to get your clothes, or even the price ranges. Can you even still shop at the same store? This is all virgin territory for you. The choices are overwhelming and honestly, you would much rather hit the gym at this point and do a few miles on the treadmill than pick through sizes and try them on. After all you got that part down pat now. Good for you!

Now you know you don't wear the same size but graze through the old selection. Not for the sizes but the names of the clothes. Now that you have a few names, move to the next smaller selection in the names you have been wearing. This is to keep you from panic, anxiety, and on course. You can only flash your panties so long before you know you have to get some pants that stays up. Today is the day!

Look through the next size down from your old size and pick one pair of pants. Then go one more size down and get another size of pants, then move to another size and get the same pair. All the same style and same color but one size smaller. Dressing rooms will let you try on 3-6 pairs of pants at one changing. When you have a selection of sizes, move to the dressing room. Time to try them on!

Start with the biggest pair of pants first. Especially if you have never worn a small size before because there will be no established memory of what you use to look like, so you have to start from scratch. First pair on and take a picture with your camera. This is to help you gauge what you look like with a second pair of eyes. Mirrors and lighting in dressing rooms can change a person's perception and may not be in your best interest but the store's interest. They want you to buy. Next, move thorough all the sizes until you find a pair that is snug around the waist and hangs correctly on the legs.

Another shocker may happen. You use to wear tall pants but now they flood the floor when you have them on. Average may not hang at the shoes. You might even find yourself…OMG!...in a pair of petites! No, you haven't shrunk in height but you have shrunk in needing extra material in the legs.

Once you have established your new size of waist (size) and length (tall, average, petite) it will be time to return to the rack and pick out different colors or different name brands. Congratulations!

Now, if you are at the half way mark and still have many pounds to lose, do not go crazy and buy a complete wardrobe yet. It will be tempting but it will be a waste of your money. If you need causal wear for work, then only pick enough pants for one week with assorted color shirts. Dresses are another way to stretch the budget in between the pounds lost because it is easy to add a belt to keep them from looking baggy and fashionable.

What is going to be the best part is looking in the mirror at home and your clothes will fit. It will be a bit of adjusting and others may notice or not but do not let that discourage your efforts. Do know that now folks will have to guess what color your panties are because your pants won't be falling down.

Passing it on

Keep a few things so you can see how far you have come in weight loss. Take pictures of your before and after.

Then pass on your things to someone who is also losing weight. This gives them support two fold. One in clothing they don't have to purchase and two motivation that they can do it too.

Perhaps even get a "lose it get it club" started at your local gym or office. Wash gently used clothing and hang them up for others to take home and wear. Savings for everyone! Everyone wins!

Types of Diets

Once you have established your food diary, reviewed your servings sizes, found your kryptonite weakness and combatted it, and now are trying to stay in x number of calories to meet your goal, what else do you want to achieve?

There are different types of diets that will help you achieve your goals.

Diabetic diets -American Diabetic Association
Diets focus on types of foods, calories allowed to keep blood sugars regulated, and offer cooking substitutes.

Heart diets- American Heart Association
Diets will focus on restricting sodium/salt and what substitutes will help keep blood pressures in check.

Arthritis- The Arthritis Foundation
Diet will focus on removing food that is high inflammation causing swelling and pain.

Ketosis
This diet focuses on restricting certain food groups to improve sugars, weight loss, and increase energy.

Everyone is on a diet. What type of food is the diet's restriction per individual? Many may need to mix several types of diets to reach their required food goals.

The Frustration of Losing Weight and the Mirror looks the Same.

One of the biggest frustrating things with losing weight is the person in the mirror looks the same. The close still fit but they may be loose. This can be very hard to deal with when there has been great success with a lot of weight lost and hard work done.

When a person is looking at losing 100 pounds or more, the mirror isn't telling the real truth of the hard work. What might work better is a tape measure. Measure the arms, legs, chest, waist, hips, and so forth. This may be a better marking of what is really going on in the mirror.

So, don't discourage. Get the tape measure out.

Measure You:

Height:

Weight:

Neck:

Chest:

Waist:

Hips:

Arms:

Legs:

Dieting Verses Life Changes Weight Loss Terminology.

There is dieting and then there is changing the way you live, eat, and types of calories you consume. Diets are types of ways you consume calories but many individuals look at types of diets as short-term events in their life to reach goals for big events. Many want to lose weight for a wedding, after a holiday, or for summer fun. The short-term goals are typically twenty pounds or less. A manageable time to restrict, exercise, or cut back on goodies that inflated the waist line that keeps us out of looking the way we wish for our life event we will be attending. This will cause individuals to go on and off diets and view them as simple controls in their eating behaviors. Individuals find that restricting from eating dessert, walking a bit more, or cutting out snacking will help them meet their goals easy.

The term dieting does not meet goals for those who want to lose more than 20 pounds in a short time frame. To the individual who needs to remove 100 pounds from their body frame, the word diet does not meet their needs. The term life style change become more of a term because it will take longer than a short term to remove 100 pounds. To remove one pound a week is 52 pounds and two pounds is 104 pounds. It may take this individual a full year of working on their body to meet the goal of 100 pounds in weight loss. Those individuals who weigh more, it may take several years to achieve their goals. This can be quite frustrating to this individual as buy it now, take it now, and see results now marketing is not going to result in the body they want now.

A life style change is just that. A change in the way life is lived to improve the body frame and lose weight. There will be some things the individual will need to change forever. A serious life style change. A different way of living, eating, and consuming calories to achieve a different body frame outlook and it may take several years of losing weight, shaping up, and maintain the weight loss. This change has to come from the individual and there will be a lot of uphill battles of temptations, failures, and others not on board with support.

No support is very hard when an individual is looking at a major hurdle of changing their life. Yet, it does come down to the individual putting their hand to their mouth. This is the person responsible. This is the person who will benefit from the change and the person who will live their new life in their new body for many more years to come. It will not be easy but it will be one of the biggest rewards this individual can do.

Recapping, a diet is typically losing weight in a short time of 20 pounds or less. A life style change is changing the way calories are consumed to lose 100 pounds are less. Those in between 20 and 100 pounds will combine both types of diet and life style change to achieve their goals.

Quick Dieting and Exercising Starts.

There are times when you are ready to go and start dieting. You already have your idea, goals, and ready to begin but just need a program. Here is a quick program to get going.

To do list:

1. Download a cell phone app for counting steps or get a tracker for your shoe to count steps.
2. Walk 30 minutes every day.
3. Stop eating anything white (food).

Why stop eating anything white? There are a couple reasons this will help with weight loss. White food tends to have more than enough carbohydrates. Carbohydrates break down into energy. Energy then needs to be stored or spent. If you are not spending your energy, you are storing it in fat rolls.

No white means no white foods; donuts, cereals, breads, pastas, snack cakes, cake, pizza crust, and so forth. You name it and it is white, no.

The advantage? Carbohydrates break down into sugars and sugars feed inflammation. This can cause arthritis to flare up and pain to increase. Cutting out white foods can cut out inflammation. More information can be found at the Arthritis Foundation website. The side effects? No pain and possible weight loss.

Another advantage to cutting out white is if a person is gluten intolerant. Gluten is typically in flour that makes all the yummy white things we love. Cut out the white and gluten is cut out too. Less stomach and intestine irritation. Another advantage is psoriasis suffers will find some relief in a gluten free diet. The side effects? Possible weight loss.

Understanding Mileage and Dieting

Great news! You picked out a diet and you have started it. Now what? Other than counting calories and monitoring your carbohydrates, fats, and proteins. What else can you do to help the number on the scale move?

Exercise! Many people do not have time or the will to do a vigorous work out but can you walk? Yes? Good? Walking is exercise and you can walk inside around the coffee table or outside around the block.

Rules of exercise: When walking, steps are counted. It roughly takes the right foot pass the left and then the right back with a left to complete a step. A number of steps equal a level of activity. A step equals to 2-2.5 feet in length. On average 2,000 steps will equal one mile. One mile can be done in a 30 minutes' walk of 3.0 mph to 3.5 mph or regular walk with no urgency. Toss in a quicker pace and 2 miles can be walked in 30 minutes.

How many steps equal what level of activity?

Sedentary steps: under 5,000 steps
Light activity: 5,000 to 7,000 steps
Active: 7,000 steps to 10,000 steps
Highly Active: 10,000 steps +

Translating steps into miles:

One mile is 2,000 steps.
Five miles is 10,000 steps.

Breaking it down to "seriously, I am walking that far?"

A 5-kilometer race is 3.1 miles or approximately 6,000+ steps.
A 10-kilometer race is 6.2 miles or approximately 12,000 steps.
A lightly active person is walking a 5K and a highly active person is walking a 10K.

To do list:

Think it cannot be done? Access a tracker to place on your shoe or download a free pedometer on your cell phone to count your steps. Walk around for two weeks to get an average of how far you are walking per day. You may be walking more than you realize and that is always a nice surprise.

Second, start adding 30 minutes of walking every day. Any time of day will do. This should be 1-2 miles depending on how fast you walk or if you add inclines to your route.

Wanting to go for glory? Needing to lose weight or training for an event…like chasing after grandchildren? Star walking 60 minutes every day. This should be about 4 miles depending on your speed.

Walking is an activity that unless you have health restrictions by a provider, this should be something everyone can do per day.

How active are you?

Sedentary steps: under 5,000 steps
Light activity: 5,000 to 7,000 steps
Active: 7,000 steps to 10,000 steps
Highly Active: 10,000 steps +

A 5-kilometer race is 3.1 miles or approximately 6,000+ steps.
A 10-kilometer race is 6.2 miles or approximately 12,000 steps.
A lightly active person is walking a 5K and a highly active person is walking a 10K.

One mile is 2,000 steps.
Five miles is 10,000 steps.

A step equals to 2-2.5 feet in length.

Passed Your Annual Exam, Now Start Diet!

The provider visit is over and you are healthy and no issues found on your exam. Time to target how much weight loss to lose and how you want to go about it. There is a realistic way to do and an unrealistic way to do it. Unrealistic ways set you up for failure, hurt feelings, and no results.

Do know that many of the fabulous bodies that are in the media and in print, did not get that way over night. Many of them took months and years to get that look. It will take time to lose weight and shape a body. Understand this is a long-term goal to look great.

Rules to the weight loss game.

1. It takes approximately 250 calories a day to lose or gain one pound a week. Two pounds per week is 500 calories per day. This means that if you ate one candy bar of 250 calories a day that by the end of the week you will gain one pound. Two candy bars a day will result in two pounds at the end of the week. To lose one pound, 250 to 500 calories must be removed per day to get the weight loss of 1-2 pounds a week.
2. Understand that the body holds fluids. Fluids are weight. There is some body weight that will not change no matter what is done to it. The body's organs and skeleton have weight and there is fluid that makes all this function and work properly. Thus, if you run out all the fluids of the body or dehydrate the body, it will lose weight. It may not continue to work properly but it will show up on the scales. This is not a true long-term weight loss. The same as emptying or cleansing the GI track. There are pounds of food that is eating that ends up in waste. The removal of waste will show up on the scales. Again, not a long-term true weight loss. The short-term weight losses that involve fluids and masses will be disappointing for long term weigh loss. Focusing on those medications or techniques long term may not result in a healthy body either.
3. Understanding what carbs or calories are. Calories break down into fats, proteins, and carbohydrates. Many diets will focus on types of foods that will follow into these categories. Eating too much of one category will have results on the scales.
4. Choosing a diet plan that meets your needs. What works well for one person may not work well for you. This is very important to understand if there is a health problem that needs to be addressed in the weight loss or weight gain program picked. IF we were all alike, one diet would work well for all of us.
5. Goals. There needs to be a goal. A goal can be short term or long term. A short-term goal is about six months or less. A long-term goal is six months or years. Thus, a short-term goal to lose weight at 1-2 pounds a week for six months will result in (1 month = 4 weeks x 6 months= 24 weeks) 24 pounds at 1-pound loss or 48 pounds in 2-pound loss. To lose 52 pounds would take 1 pound a week for a year or 2 pounds a year would equal 104 pounds. Understanding it is going to take time to lose weight will keep you from failing. Do know that the time is going to pass anyway. You will weigh less or you will not. Your choice.
6. Responsibility. You are the one who puts food in your mouth. It is your choice what you eat, when you eat, and what you eat. Just because the mountain is there does not mean you have to climb it.

Annual Well Check Up Before Diets

One of the necessary things before starting a diet is to go to your provider and get a head to toe assessment and laboratory work up. Be sure your version of healthy is really healthy or not. This visit will include your vital signs, body mass index (BMI), and chemical blood work. This will show if there are problems with blood pressure, BMI, and any chemical problems with your thyroid, kidneys, and possible diabetes.

Why is this so important? Mainly because it will keep you from failing at your weight loss efforts. It will give you a realistic idea of where you are in the human "normal" and not the photoshop version of human. You may be surprised that your BMI is in the normal range. You may not need to lose weight but you may need to tone the body. This means that the shift from losing weight to the shift of exercise is more important. The type of exercises that will need to be done to get the idea of what body should be looking back from the mirror, may mean exercises like planks, squats, and weight lifts. This will mean a different diet. Not one to lose weight but one to help build muscle.

Other problems found may be too high blood pressure, blood sugars, and a chemical imbalance in the blood. This will set you on a different type of diet. The wrong diet can cause your health to be worse, not better. Finding out there is a health problem will help pick out the right diet to follow. Often, just adjusting the diet and calorie intake to lower blood pressure and correct blood sugars will result in weight loss. Finding out there is a thyroid problem and starting medication can result in weight loss or weight gain.

To do list:

1. Visit your provider for a well checkup or annual visit. At this visit discuss your health and get your laboratory work done to see if you are "normal" or have health issues that is derailing your diet efforts.
2. Finding out you are "normal" range for your height and weight is a body mass index (BMI). This means that you may start shaping your body. Time to review exercise plans, cardio to weigh lifting on how to get the image desired.
3. Finding out there is a health problem. First, addressing the health problem. Eating to get the blood pressure or blood sugar in range. Starting any medications and keeping them monitored to achieve a "normal". Adjusting any weight loss or weight gaining efforts with regular visits to the provider to keep you on track.
4. You are healthy and no issues found on your exam. Time to target how much weight loss to lose and how you want to go about it.

Deciding to lose weight?

It happens to everyone once in a while. Looking into the mirror and deciding that you do not like the image looking back. The image has way too much extra around the middle. Clothes do not hang right or way too tight. It may even happen when you find you cannot do the things you use to do or maybe you never could do those things and you want to do them, sort of check of that bucket list of achievements.

Next is how do you do it? There is an assortment of weight loss ideas to choose from but the best thing you can do first is be honest with yourself. What are your bad habits? Too much beverage out of the vending machine? Too many party drinks over the weekend? Eating out all the time and picking the highest carb loaded food you can order?

Where do you even start if you do not even know what you are doing wrong? What if you have been doing some exercise and eating healthy foods? Where are you going wrong? Or you going wrong? Something is not happening to make the person in the mirror not look the way you wish. Are you being realistic in your ideas? Do you have a real idea what folks look like and live in a non-photoshop world?
Time to check the reality of where you stand and looking back from the mirror.

1. Go to your provider and get a head to toe assessment and laboratory work up. Be sure your version of healthy is really healthy or not. This visit will include your vital signs, body mass index (BMI), and chemical blood work. This will show if there are problems with blood pressure, BMI, and any chemical problems with your thyroid, kidneys, and possible diabetes.
2. Next, data log all the food eaten every day for two weeks. No dieting, just getting an idea what you really are eating and if it is healthy or not. You may be in for some surprises. You may be eating healthy but the portion size, condiment, or extras have hidden calories that make the meal higher in carbs than you thought. You may find that you are just eating way too much in a day or one meal is blowing your entire efforts of weight loss. There are several ways to log your meals, on paper or digital. No wrong way, just begin and keep logging all the food and drinks consumed.
3. Exercise totals. All movement is exercise in some way but one of the easiest ways to log exercise is walking and how many steps are taken. Again, any counter that is automatic and applies to your shoe or a digital app for your cell will work. Use it and start your counting. Get an idea how many steps you are doing in one day. You may already be doing a lot more steps that you thought you were doing.

This is to get what is known in the medical world as a baseline. This baseline will be what your future efforts will be compared too. You can start right now. No need to wait for a special day to begin. You are just trying to get a baseline of what your health is right now.

To do list:

1. Make an appointment for a well visit check up with laboratory work to be done.
2. Start logging all your food and drinks for two weeks.
3. Log all steps and exercise for two weeks.

Laboratory Work Up

Hemoglobin Alc –diabetic

Cholesterol- heart disease

Vitamin D3 – bone weakness

Hemoglobin/Hemocrit- anemia

TSH- thyroid

Glucose- blood sugar

WBC – white blood cells/infections or inflammation

Hormones- pregnancy, menopause or low testosterone levels

And more...

Ten Ways the Doctor Told You to Lose Weight, Not.

When you make an appointment with a provider, weight may come up. Not a terrible problem as most folks are pretty aware that the scales cried when they stepped on it. What was hurtful was when the provider stated to lose weight but didn't say how.
Why do they do this? As a provider, I can answer this.

1. The provider didn't schedule time to talk about weight. They just noticed it on the vital sign sheet that it was not in the normal range. They need to say something because it isn't in the normal range. Same as if your blood pressure is too high. Your weight is high. You need to lose weight.
2. They didn't say how to lose weight. They may be on a crunch system of needing to see so many patients per hour and they were behind before they clocked in for the day. They can only discuss what you came in to be seen for and only that or they will be in the office forever.
3. They don't have time to school you on nutrition but they might have time to refer you to a dietitian.
4. They don't know what you have tried and may not be able to offer you a diet pill. Many want a diet pill and while they will cause you to lose weight, your other health problems may prevent it from working for you. There may even be a law in your state that stops those types of medications from getting prescribed as they are abused.
5. Do you know what exercise means? Often, it is assumed you don't. You may really be trying hard and walking everywhere but the weight is hanging on you. What else could you do?
6. You have a health problem that is stopping you from losing weight. Ask your provider to check your blood work to rule this out.
7. This isn't their specialty. They don't consider themselves a diet clinic and don't want to mess with it or really don't have extensive knowledge in weight loss, what works, and what won't.
8. They think you want a quick answer and quick result. Maybe you are fully aware that your weight didn't happen overnight. You gained weight over your marriage or university career. Now what should you do?
9. Motivation is necessary. Maybe you have been ignoring the weight and they may think calling you out on your weight will make you motivated to do something. When God talks to you, you listen right? So, they are telling you, do something about it.
10. You leave hurt and angry. Don't do that. Before you leave the office, book another appointment to discuss your weight or get a referral to someone who can. Maybe the next appointment will be filled with all the information you needed that you may earn yourself an honorary degree on dieting the next time you visit. You won't know if you don't set up a follow up appointment.

Do know that understanding you are overweight is the first step in moving toward fixing the problem. Finding out what your body mass index (BMI) should be verses what it is, should be noted on that "you need to lose weight" announcement.

Weight Loss and Mental Health Changes in Body

One of the biggest mistakes of losing weight is that it will change your mental health. It may not. What weight loss will do is change how others may treat you based on how you weigh. There are all types of discrimination but discrimination on weight happens a lot more than many realize. Mainly because there is a standard to everything. The standard size bed, chair, door, and room. If you are the standard weight, then those standard things will fit you just fine. If you are not the standard size then things won't fit you. Accommodations will need to be made for you and those accommodations may not be mandatory or mandated they have to be.

Same can be said with mental health. How you see yourself, your self-respect, your self-worth, and chemical changes in the brain may not change with weight loss. Coping skills that were never there before weight loss may not be there after weight loss. You will have to develop these missing coping skills and may or not have changes in medications to get the effect needed. Weight loss may not cure your mental health problems.

This is when talking with a provider before weight loss may be necessary regarding changings in mental health medications. Regular monthly checkups may be necessary with a mental health provider as you move forward with weight loss. Having a mental health specialist to help guide and adjust medications as you lose weight may be beneficial. It will help with creating new coping skills or establishing coping skills.

Joining a support group of folks going through weight loss programs, changes, or directed programs with surgical weight loss programs may be very beneficial post dramatic weight loss. Mental health is something everyone has and it may be good, bad, or in need of help by talking with someone to needing medications to feel "normal". It is not as taboo as many use to think. Our world is always changing and living in it requires constant challenges that not all of us having coping skills to deal with and sometimes we need help. This is okay. This is normal to ask for help.

How Did You Lose the Weight?

Newly thin or dieting folks get this question a lot. Nearly everyone will ask how you did it. Losing weight is a struggle for everyone and not everyone is motivated to start or many want a new way to try that might be easy or work for them.

First up, there is no easy. Weight loss or weight gain does not happen overnight unless you have a disease like congestive heart failure where you can put on 10 pounds over night in body water. There is no losing a great amount of weight in a week either. You can dehydrate your body to lose several pounds or laxative city to clean out the GI. Both will show fluid loss on the scales. Not necessarily a healthy thing to do and nor should you. Unless you are getting ready for a colonoscopy, then laxative away. You don't want to repeat this event.

Second up, it can be very upsetting to think others thought you did this easy and quickly. You didn't. It can take months to years to get the body you wish. Many who do weight loss surgery have to prep 6 months to a year before surgery to be ready. This is then followed by months up to a year of losing weight. It may mean more surgeries, gym time, and changes in eating the same way every day. It wasn't an easy way to do it to get the results. Don't be fooled into thinking it was or is.

Third, many may even correct you on how you did it or not believe what you are saying is true. What do you mean you just cut back? Why, do they do this? Because the already tried this and it didn't work for them, so why would it work for you?

Do they really want to know how you did it? There may be a few folks looking for support or a place to start. Will the diet work for them? Maybe or not, depends on their efforts, not your efforts. That is the part they may not want to believe.

So, what do you say to someone who ask? Because they will ask you. Many don't want to hear a play by play on how you did it unless you are selling a product or something to them. Thus, give them a standard sentence of "I go to the gym." Or "I only eat 1500 calories per day." It gives them a focus and they will either be satisfied with the answer or ask a few more questions on how. Mainly they are looking for motivation and help from you. It will be up to you if you want to be supportive or not.

Surprising Weight Loss Changes

There are a lot of things that you will not be prepared for when you lose weight. Mainly because you aren't thinking or realize these things will happen to you. These are going to be the things that you will get tickled about with your new weight loss that many may not understand unless they also when through such a change.

Things that may surprise you now:

Crossing your legs. Yes, you can do that now. Before there was so much weight on your legs that was not even possible. You will become amazed at being able to do this. You may want to wear underwear in the company of others as things are more noticeable now.

Fitting into a booth next time you eat out. You have always requested a table with chairs. Now you can sit in a booth with your arms down at your sides. No arms on the table now. You may even have lost so much weight that someone can sit next to you on your side of the booth!

Freaking out because you are now the size as the general public. Before when you went shopping XXXXL shirt would be there when you went back to get it. Now you are the same size as a good percentage of the population and that shirt will be gone now. When you see it, you have to get it, or you want be able to get it.

Temperature changes. Remember when you would turn up the A/C so you wouldn't sweat? Now that same choice of temperature has you wrapping up with a blanket. Losing the extra body weight equaled body heat. Not all bad. Suddenly, hanging out side in the sun doesn't melt you like ice cream on a hot day. You actually want to spend time outside now. You may hardly even sweat at some of the things that use to make you sweat and save countries from droughts from the excess water you produced. You may even get it why girls get those long sleeves to cover up their fingers. You are a bit colder now. Holy Moley! You want to own all the sweaters now when you were strictly just a tee shirt in the winter.

Body cleaning products. Where did all the soap come from? Same dab won't do you anymore. Soap is everywhere now. Things you use to lather with in great quantities are over the top now. Don't buy anything you really are okay with because it is going to last longer. Think, can you deal with pumpkin spice in the spring? Wait there is more! This huge bath tub you own! Did elves come in and change it out? You now have room beside your body with water all around you! Those with jet tubs are going to find they can swim laps! Who would of thought?

Body parts not in the way. This can be very exciting to not have to move extra rolls to get to things that need to be cleaned. Before it would make showering longer because you broke out in sweat just trying to clean everything. Not anymore. Zip, zip, and you are now done.

Towels are bigger. You can put a towel around you now. Before it only covered the front and you walked size ways through the house to get your clothes, trying to hide your back side. Now you can change into your clothes in the bathroom with no fear of falling or getting those clothes wet. No extra drying time needed now.

Storage is more. That XXXL sweater took up the entire drawer it was in or most of the closet storage. Not anymore! Where did all that space come from? Like, when did you get a walk-in closet?
Space now equals space! Chairs and beds that use to be too small are now huge to you. It does take a while to get use to the change but go you!

Pretty neat things you won't realize until you have lost weight. Things you didn't know you would notice and now you get tickled about the changes.

Note:

The US did away with standard size clothes in 1985. The standards are based on body mass index (BMI) and each size correlated with a BMI.

Plus size has changed to mean that smaller sizes are now plus size but those clothes did not change in size, just the labels.

Do not get caught up in wearing a particular size. If you ask a fashion designer to make you a size 4 they will make you a size 4 but it will be on the label not the actual outfit.

The other thing to consider is the population is taller and wider in general than prior times. This is due to the changes of the chemicals in food, along with better health care.

Scary Response to Weight Loss Changes

There are things we don't talk about when we lose weight because we are focused on losing the weight. When you are grossly obese, fat, and overweight most of your life, you don't know a lot of things that skinny, thin, and folks in the right size all their life know.

There is a huge learning curve on behaviors and changes in behaviors. This can be quite startling, distracting, and even frightening to those who do lose weight loss.

We focus on the weight loss and not the emotional responses from others. This can be terrifying depending on the results to some.

Here are some changes that you will notice on a long weight loss journey. This is someone who has never experienced "thin" and it can cause folks to second guess their choice and regain weight.

Everyone treats you different now. Not just looking at you because you are thin but may take it on another level by talking to you, when prior they wouldn't give you the time of day, to aggressively wanting to touch you or trying to pick you up, followed by carrying you off. This is very shocking to a newly thin person. Remember no is no. Touch and picking you up is no. The person inside is still the person with less weight on their body. This does not mean they can be touched. It also means you are assaulting them. Touching another person with no person is assault. Period.

Self-defense becomes necessary for the newly thin person. Especially since safety for a fat person isn't as much of a high priority because very few fat folks get kidnapped. Fat people know they are safer and tend to not have safety as a priority always in the forethought of their minds. The 2 am trip to get ice cream is no big deal. It becomes a big deal when you are thinner. You weigh less and you can be knocked over, picked up, and carried off.

Carrying a concealed weapon (CCW) becomes a concern with women who lose weight quickly and are drawing men and women out of the woodworks. Some folks may even find they have stalkers. Very terrifying and newly thin person may even find they don't want to leave their homes because of this new fear. A CCW gives them a support system they didn't know they needed until they were thin. The extra person was the fat they lost. That person isn't there anymore.

Assertiveness becomes necessary. Many folks will say she use to be so sweet when she was fat. Now she isn't. She may have accepted she couldn't change anything that was said before and let a lot of things roll off her shoulders that now she no longer has to put up with. Working 24/7 to lose weight, helps one to build up some courage and angry that use to be hushed, is now released. She was assertive in needing to go to the gym, not eat everything in the refrigerator, and tell you no with meaning, is just that, no. She is not responsible for your feelings, you are. She is not the problem now, you are.

Losing a lot of weight is just the beginning for how the person inside is changing. Just because they are skinny now does not mean they will say yes to you, want to date you, or find you more attractive. They remember how you treated them when they were fat, told them no, and didn't ask them out. That person inside didn't change. You did.

Recommended at any weight or age:

- Defense classes
- Safety classes
- CPR
- Basic Life Support
- Reviewing and knowing your current local, state, and country laws
- First aid classes
- Swimming classes
- Driving classes
- CCW classes (even if you choose not to carry/own a gun)
- Cooking classes
- Fire safety classes
- Voting registration

Did you enjoy this book? Excellent! *Do You Know Lisa, Volume 5* is just around the corner!

Coming soon! The weight loss of Team Goins, how they lost all that weight! Watch for the book and videos to come out in 2018!

"Ideas are easy. It is implementing them that is the hard part."

~Dr. Lisa Goins PhD, APRN, FNP-BC, RMT

9 781979 078924